T0256249

The International Library of Psychology

HINDU PSYCHOLOGY

Founded by C. K. Ogden

The International Library of Psychology

PSYCHOLOGY AND RELIGION
In 6 Volumes

HINDU PSYCHOLOGY

Its Meaning for the West

SWAMI AKHILANANDA

Introduction by Gordon W Allport

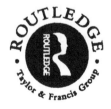

First published in 1948
by Routledge

Reprinted in 1999, 2000
by Routledge
2 Park Square, Milton Park, Abingdon, Oxfordshire OX14 4RN
711 Third Avenue, New York, NY 10017

First issued in paperback 2014

Routledge is an imprint of the Taylor and Francis Group, an informa business

Transferred to Digital Printing 2007

British Library Cataloguing in Publication Data
A CIP catalogue record for this book
is available from the British Library

Hindu Psychology
ISBN 978-0-415-21110-9 (hbk)
ISBN 978-1-138-00741-3 (pbk)
Psychology and Religion: 6 Volumes
ISBN 978-0-415-21133-8
The International Library of Psychology: 204 Volumes
ISBN 978-0-415-19132-6

Table of Contents

Introduction

IT IS inexcusable that we who think in the Western frame of thought should be as ignorant as we are of the frame of thought of the East. Year after year we have spent our time thinking exclusively in the thought forms of our own Western culture, in practicing or examining the tradition of our own religion, and in evolving our own Western theories of the mind. Few of us have spent even one day of our lives learning about the thought forms that control the minds of millions of our fellow men who adhere to the basic religion of Hinduism. Since in modern days we can no longer deny that all mankind lives in One World, such ignorance of our Eastern cousin's mind is as dangerous as it is inexcusable.

Does the excited psychology of action and behavior so characteristic of America treat adequately all the capacities of the human mind? Are the powers of meditation revealed through *yoga* illusory and slightly absurd? Is it conceivable that the energies released through mental discipline are of no potential use to men who live in the West? Ignorance of Eastern thought leads us to give callow and mischievous answers to such questions as these.

Swami Akhilananda makes available to us a nontechnical introduction to the thought of the East. He does so in a direct and lucid style. Understanding and appreciating the significance of much of Western psychology, he is able to point shrewdly to certain improvements that Eastern psychology can offer, and to chasms it may help to fill. At the same time he stresses in a manner agreeable to Americans the applications of Hindu psychology. In this respect he shows that he sympathizes with the pragmatic interest of Americans. He is an architect bent on building a bridge between hemispheres.

I do not mean to say that complete co-ordination between Hindu and American psychology will be easily achieved. In some respects, I am convinced, American psychology would improve in richness and wisdom if it accommodated in some way the wise things that the author says about meditation and the necessity for an adequate philosophy of life. In respect to the more occult manifestations of mental powers to which he occasionally refers, I am not so certain. Whether the occult element in Hindu psychology stems from its relative lack of acquaintance with what we in the West call "scientific method," or whether this Western "scientific method" is nothing but a narrow cult that blinds itself to uncongenial phenomena, I am not at this moment prepared to say. Perhaps concessions are needed on both sides.

But the problem of the occult plays a minor role in this book. From the author I have learned, as others will, many basic facts about the thought forms of the Hindu religion and the Hindu direction of mental life. Such knowledge is intrinsically rewarding. It is also timely since it helps build for the coming era needed bridges between great families of the human race.

GORDON W. ALLPORT
Psychology Department
Harvard University

Foreword

ALL too many there are who quote Rudyard Kipling's famous lines (often stopping with the first line):

> Oh, East is East, and West is West, and never the twain shall meet.
> Till Earth and Sky stand presently at God's great Judgment Seat.

All too few remember how Kipling continued:

> But there is neither East nor West, Border, nor Breed, nor Birth,
> When two strong men stand face to face, though they come from the ends of the earth!

The spirit can triumph over geography and race. Kipling's restriction of the spirit of universality to "strong men" is, we must grant, too individualistic, too aristocratic and Nietzschean to lead the world on the path to spiritual unity. Yet humanity has a long way to go before it fulfills Kipling's vision of "neither East nor West, Border, nor Breed, nor Birth."

Too many Occidentals judge the East entirely in terms of its economic poverty, human suffering, caste distinctions, and social maladjustments. Too many Orientals judge the West entirely in terms of its exploitation of less favored races, its materialistic love of profit and comfort, its disloyalty to religion, and its ruthless and suicidal warfare. All races and regions will be condemned when only their weaknesses and sins are considered. All races and regions will be appreciated when their highest achievements and possibilities are taken into account.

It is fortunate for the United States that so many worthy representatives of other cultures come to live in this country and to share their thought with Americans. Notable among these valued guests is the Swami Akhilananda, who for some years has been conducting worship and instruction in the Ramakrishna Vedanta Centers of Providence, Rhode Island, and Boston, Massachusetts. He has made many friends in educational circles, especially at Brown, Boston, and Harvard Universities. He is welcome among Jews and Christians alike. He is prized both as a scholar and as a religious leader and counselor.

It is a great privilege for me to be counted among the friends of this broad-minded and noble man. He is modest, gentle, and tolerant; yet at the same time firm, well-poised, and saintly. In this book he has set forth some of the psychological principles of the art of living. The reader may be assured that the Swami lives by the principles which he here recommends to others. He may also be assured that the purpose of this book is not to lead him to substitute Indian psychology for Christianity or Judaism. The Swami esteems these religions highly. Not only does his Vedanta faith forbid him to speak evil of any religion, but also it leads him to acknowledge the presence of divine reality in every religion. The principles which the Swami Akhilananda sets forth in this book are universal, not sectarian. They are based on the results of centuries of experience and spiritual experiment as truly as science is based on the work of centuries of physical experiment.

There is a sense in which his insights represent both the oldest and the youngest Hindu wisdom. The oldest, because all Indian devotees are students of the ancient scriptures of the Vedas and Upanishads, and of commentators and philosophers who have interpreted the spiritual principles of Hinduism; and the youngest, because the faith which he represents is an outgrowth of the teaching and religious experience of Sri Ramakrishna, a nineteenth-century saint, whose immediate disciple, the Swami Brahmananda, was the teacher of the Swami Akhilananda. To know our author, then, is analogous to knowing one of the early Christians who was separated from Jesus by only one generation.

These facts may serve to explain the combination of maturity and vitality, of theoretical insight and practical sense, which one finds in this book. The reader may approach it with any faith or with no faith. Let him read it with open mind. Few indeed will be those who study it and try even a few of its suggestions without experiencing some new calm, peace, and strength in the inner life.

East and West need each other. Each is richer in some goods, poorer in others. The West cannot afford to neglect the gifts which wise men from the East may bring.

EDGAR SHEFFIELD BRIGHTMAN
Philosophy Department
Boston University

Preface

THE various chapters of this book were originally given as extemporaneous lectures in Boston and Providence. Some friends were anxious to have a record of these lectures and employed stenographers to take notes on them. At that time it was not definitely known whether they would form the chapters of a book or not. However, as the lectures were received enthusiastically by the audiences, our friends were anxious to have a permanent record. Our late friend, Dr. Raymond Willoughby, formerly of Brown University, attended some of the lectures and read the notes. He told us: "You [Hindus] have something to give us for the training of the mind." So the lectures were edited and elaborated for publication in book form.

Historical treatment of the development of the science of psychology in India has not been attempted. This book rather gives an idea of the achievement of the science of psychology by both Hindus and Buddhists in India. It also offers the methods that are adopted in India to develop the mind itself. It may seem that more elaborate treatment and historical development should be given in a book on Hindu psychology, as there is no work on this subject so far as we know.

This book is presented to both Eastern and Western readers to stimulate their interest in the achievements of the Hindus in the science of psychology. It is given in brief form, as the majority of the people are too busy to spend much of their time in reading. Our suggestion to Eastern scholars is that they be prepared to share their knowledge with Western thinkers and readers. They should contribute unhesitatingly and unsparingly what they can give to the West in the fields of religion, psychology, and philosophy. On the other hand, they should be prepared to receive what the West can contribute in the field of science and other forms of discipline. Our request to Western readers and thinkers is that they use the achievements of India in the field of psychology. It will be extremely gratifying if interest can be created in the readers so that they will further study and practice the Hindu system of psychology. Their efforts will considerably lessen mutual mistrust, suspicion, and misunderstanding and will bring a great deal of benefit to all groups of people in the world.

It should be mentioned that Hindu psychology includes both Hindu and Buddhistic systems of thought and methods of psychology. They have comingled so much in India ever since the fifth century B.C. that it would be impossible to separate them. Both Hindu and Buddhistic psychologists use many methods in common for mental development.

Often Western thinkers consider Hindu philosophy and psychology something mysterious; consequently, they almost neglect to mention it in their historic treatment of these branches of knowledge. It is our conviction that this is due to the Western scholars' lack of knowledge of the Hindu schools of thought. Unfortunately, the word *yoga* almost invariably arouses curiosity and suspicion in the West. We have tried to dispel the confused notions of Western readers. Hindu psychology and the systems of *yoga* are neither mysterious, suspicious, nor amusing. They are based on thorough scientific methods of observation and experiment.

The first two chapters of this book may seem to be technical and uninteresting from the "pragmatic" point of view. It was necessary to give a complete picture of the mind as conceived by Hindu psychologists, so we had to run the risk of making the treatment a little technical as a basis for the understanding of perception and knowledge. Therefore, readers are requested to continue with patience until they reach the practical aspects of Hindu psychology and its value in life.

The credit for this book goes completely to the teachings, love, blessings, and inspiration of our beloved Master, Swami Brahmananda, and to our beloved leader, Swami Vivekananda, two great disciples of Sri Ramakrishna. We must mention the name of Swami Premananda, another great disciple of Sri Ramakrishna, who is considerably responsible for our humble contribution, as he used to insist on our study of scientific methods. We are also humbly grateful to other disciples of Sri Ramakrishna for their ideals and lives and for their loving blessings to us.

The manuscript was read wholly or partly by all the Swamis of the Ramakrishna Order in America. Swami Bodhananda of New York, Swami Prabhavananda of Los Angeles, and Swami Vishwananda of Chicago should be especially mentioned for their constant encouragement. Our good friends Professor Edgar S. Brightman of Boston University, Professor Gordon W. Allport of Harvard University, Professor Paul E. Johnson of Boston University, Professor Joachim Wach of Brown University, Professor Parry Moon of the Massachusetts Institute of Technology, and Professor Orval Hobart Mowrer of Harvard University kindly read the manuscript and gave valuable suggestions. We are especially grateful to Professor Brightman and Professor Allport for writing the Foreword and Introduction as well as for their interest in the publication of the book. We are also indebted to some of our students and friends who arranged for stenographers, typed the manuscript, and helped in other ways. We also thankfully acknowledge the authors and publishers who kindly and graciously permitted their books to be quoted.

We offer the result of this humble effort to the All Loving Being.

AKHILANANDA

Vedanta Society
Boston, Massachusetts
November 12, 1945

HINDU PSYCHOLOGY

ITS MEANING
FOR THE WEST

CHAPTER I

A Survey of Western and Hindu Psychology

YEARS ago, the psychology of the classical schools in the West was concerned chiefly with the study of the mind in its successive states of awareness. The older psychologists described the functionings of the mind, observed how it behaved, and then tried to discover the laws that governed its activities. However, these studies were always limited to the conscious plane. We seldom find any reference to the study of other mental aspects. Even the great psychologist, Wundt, as well as other notable persons in the field, seemed unaware of the activities of the hidden states of mind now known as the subconscious or unconscious. Although psychologists formed different schools of thought according to their various theories of the subjective and objective elements of consciousness and the relation of these elements to the physical body, they all studied the conscious elements only, ignoring the subconscious and superconscious states of mind. From their observations, many of them came to the conclusion that consciousness and soul had no existence separate from physical brain matter and that they were really only products of brain matter. Materialistic thinkers completely ignored the fact that there could be a separate existence of mind or consciousness, to say nothing of a separate existence of the soul, although Wundt and his followers expounded psychophysical parallelism.

It is true that the mind usually functions in ordinary

persons through the nervous system and brain cells, just as electricity functions and is manifested through wires and electrical apparatus.[1] Yet one cannot conclude that the electricity and the wires are identical. Similarly, the mind in its functionings, conscious or otherwise, cannot be identified with the instruments through which it works or has expression.

The trend of modern science, however, is in a direction different from that taken by the materialists of the last century. Some of the modern scientists, unlike their predecessors, are not dogmatic in their views. We do not wish to imply that the psychologists of the older schools of thought were the only ones to put forth their ideas as ultimate solutions. Physicists, chemists, and general scientists were also dogmatic and tenacious in their opinions. Today it is a pleasure to find that some of the greatest thinkers, some of the most notable psychologists, are taking a liberal stand. They do not limit themselves to one aspect of a subject but are ready to regard it from other points of view, always keeping themselves open to conviction. Many of them are willing to concede that the mind may continue to exist after the dissolution of the body and brain. Dr. William Brown, one of the outstanding psychologists and psychiatrists of Europe, is much inclined to accept the theory of the post-existence of the mind. The evidence which he himself has gathered, and which was obtained for him from authoritative sources upon which he could depend, has convinced him that there is a strong possibility of the continued existence of the mind after the death of the physical body. He says:

It would not be easy to define the scope of psychical research, but we may perhaps state as its most characteristic problem . . .

[1] In Chapters IX and X we shall see, in the cases of extrasensory perceptions and superconsciousness which are cited, that the mind can function without the help of the nervous system as an instrument of perception.

how far the embodied mind can get into communication with disembodied minds, the minds of those who have already died, the minds that are to be presumed, either on the authority of religion or on the basis of fact, to be still existing elsewhere than in visible human form on this planet.[2]

Professor Eddington says in his discussion of science and mysticism:

We have seen that the cyclic scheme of physics presupposes a background outside the scope of its investigations. In this background we must find first, our own personality, and then perhaps a greater personality. The idea of a universal Mind or Logos would be, I think, a fairly plausible inference from the present state of scientific theory, at least it is in harmony with it.[3]

Again, Dr. Richard Müller-Freienfels of Germany, in *Evolution of Modern Psychology*, does not discard certain mental experiences which have no sense element in them, but he suggests that they be subjected to scientific investigation.[4] Such frank statements coming from psychologists and other scientists clearly show a definite tendency to differ from and even to refute the theories of the materialists of the last century. The opinions of Professor Gordon W. Allport, Sir Oliver Lodge, Dr. Alexis Carrel, and Dr. Gustaf Stromberg, author of *The Soul of the Universe*,[5] are also included with this group of thinkers.

It is interesting to note that psychology itself is no longer limited to the study of the conscious mental plane, and careful analyses of the activities of the subconscious state

[2] William Brown, *Science and Personality* (Oxford University Press. 1929), p. 183.

[3] A. S. Eddington, *Nature of the Physical World* (Cambridge University Press, 1928), p. 338.

[4] Richard Müller-Freienfels, *Evolution of Modern Psychology*, trans. W. Béran Wolfe (New Haven: Yale University Press, 1935).

[5] Gustaf Stromberg, *The Soul of the Universe* (Philadelphia: David McKay Co., 1940).

are being made. This alone is a wonderful achievement and a great advance in the field of mental science. Of course, exceptions to this are found in the behaviorists, reflexologists, and other mechanistic psychologists who reject not only the subconscious but also the conscious states. Even these thinkers by their denials show that these mental states cannot be ignored and that there are certain phenomena which must be satisfactorily explained somehow if we are to understand the human personality.

Psychoanalysis has made amazing strides in this modern age. The experiments performed and the evidence gathered are really surprising. In their attempts to obtain a clear understanding of the activities that are going on beneath the surface of the conscious plane, psychologists are making definite and deliberate experiments upon the hidden mind. They are analyzing carefully the different psychological states and mental functionings. This is difficult because they are dealing with subtle and elusive mental forces that cannot be easily apprehended. These forces are often not reducible to scientific formulas nor subject to conclusive proof. Anyone can study or observe certain psychological states and processes that are going on in the conscious plane, but it requires penetrating analytical intelligence, intuitive insight, clarity of vision, and the utmost patience to try to grasp the functionings of the hidden states of the subconscious aspect of the mind. Often one has only inference upon which to depend. People behave in certain ways; they have certain reactions. From observation of their conduct and study of their habits the psychoanalyst tries to discover the root from which their actions spring—the motivating cause of their behavior. This is to be found within the subconscious mind.

Nowadays, most of the dynamic psychologists of the West —except, of course, the behaviorists and others of similar type—believe that man's behavior and many of his conscious activities are really determined by the subconscious mind. For instance, if you have any kind of fear they will not leave you alone until they have discovered the underlying cause. They want to know why you have that fear and what is in your subconscious state that produces it. Similarly, they will analyze other tendencies, too, until they are satisfied that they have found the root of the mental difficulty and can explain why you are reacting in this or that manner.

According to Freud, Jung, and others, the greater portion of the mind is actually submerged, unknown to every one of us. Hindus agree with them in this respect. The mind can be compared to an iceberg. Although only a small portion is visible above the water, nevertheless the submerged part of it exists and is a power to be reckoned with. From the surface of the water one cannot easily gauge the size of the whole iceberg, yet it may be powerful enough to destroy a huge ship such as the ill-fated "Titanic." Similarly, the submerged mind, the subconscious state, is a potent factor and powerful enough to determine even conscious tendencies. Often we do not realize what influences are hidden there. A man may not be aware of the forces that lie beneath the surface of his mind, nor can these forces be suspected by an untrained observer. Hindu psychologists call these hidden mental forces *samskaras.*[6]

Modern psychology has developed another aspect of the study of the mind that is a unique contribution to the Western world, especially to medical science. The greater number of our diseases are now believed to be functional and caused by maladjustment, conflict, frustration, or lack of mental balance with consequent disorder of the nervous system. This may be a surprise to many persons. How can

[6] *Raja Yoga* by Swami Vivekananda and the *Yoga Aphorisms of Patanjali* are recommended for further study of the Hindu point of view.

this be? How can the mind and nerves affect the body in such a way as to cause organic disease?

When the nerves do not function properly, ailments appear in certain organs. Psychologists tell us that many of the so-called organic diseases had their beginning when the organs could not function properly owing to mental maladjustments, conflict, and consequent lack of balance in the nervous system. We all know that the nervous system plays a vital and most important part in our lives. It is closely connected with the mind and is easily affected by the slightest mental disorder. Therefore, mental troubles which are reflected in the nervous system can be shown as the real cause of many functional diseases. Also many cases of insanity, neuroses and psychoses, can be traced to mental dissatisfaction and agitation, frustration and conflict.

A few years ago at an annual conference regarding medical education, eminent medical men expressed their strong belief that students of medicine should study psychiatry and that the degree of Doctor of Medicine should include requirements for an understanding of analytical psychology.[7] This shows definitely that modern medical science is taking into consideration the mental condition of a patient, and significance is being given to the effect of the mind on the body. Psychosomatic treatment is advocated by Dr. Franz Alexander in *The Medical Value of Psychoanalysis*.[8] This

---

[7] "The Importance of Introducing Psychiatry into General Internship," *Journal of the American Medical Association*, CII (1934), 982-86 and 1231-32. The late Dean A. S. Begg of Boston University introduced the study of the nervous system in the first year of medical school, followed by physiology and its bearing on the nervous system. In the second year, neuropathology and psychiatric principles were introduced. According to Dr. E. S. Ryerson of Toronto University, the study of psychology was compulsory in the second year of medical school. Dr. C. C. Burlingame of Hartford, Connecticut, and Dr. Franklin Ebaugh recommended a knowledge of fundamental psychiatry during internship.

[8] Franz Alexander, *The Medical Value of Psychoanalysis* (London: Allen and Unwin, 1936), chaps. V and VI.

book and Dr. Carl Binger's *The Doctor's Job* are very helpful for reference.[9]

The motivating forces behind man's activities are being
seriously studied by modern psychologists, but there are
points of difference between the Eastern and Western schools
of thought. The Hindu psychologists agree that man has
various urges and instincts, but they do not accept the theories of Freud and Adler that either the sex urge or the will
to power is the most predominant instinct or that it is the
fundamental truth of man's nature. In this connection, the
ideas of Dr. William Brown resemble those of the Hindu
psychologists because he holds that neither sex nor the will
to power is enough to explain human behavior and action.
Dr. Brown also comments, in *Science and Personality*, that
although Freud and Adler tried to discover one predominant
instinct in man they have failed.

Freud later seemed to change from his theory of one basic
urge of sex (pleasure) to a theory of two basic urges—"life
instinct" and "death instinct," or sex urge and suicide urge.
He evidently concluded that these two are not mutually exclusive urges in man; they intermingle in human behavior.
According to him and some of his followers, such as Dr.
Karl A. Menninger, author of *Man Against Himself*,[10] life
is a struggle between these two forces.

Hindu psychologists do not agree with the view that man
has a basic destructive tendency. Suicide, war, and all other
such destructive tendencies are not expressions of the normal
mind. It seems that Freud and other psychoanalysts make
unnecessary and uncalled-for generalizations from the study
of pathological cases. It is also equally illogical and superficial to trace the death or destructive urge even in religious

[9] Carl Binger, *The Doctor's Job* (New York: W. W. Norton & Co., Inc., 1945),
chap. VIII.
[10] Karl A. Menninger, *Man Against Himself* (London: Harrap, 1938).

self-abnegation and sacrifice. An unbiased understanding of the true spirit of religious culture will convince us that Freudian conclusions of this sort are thoroughly unjustified. The view of the Hindu psychologists is just the opposite. They come to the conclusion that there is an urge for eternal happiness and eternal existence in the human mind. The search after abiding happiness, bliss, is the real motive power behind man's activities both conscious and unconscious, as Spinoza affirmed. The tendency to destruction, or the suicide urge, is not the basic and inherent quality of man; hatred, war, and other destructive activities are rather due to the perverted application and erroneous understanding of this urge for happiness.

Dr. William McDougall also differs from the Freudian and Adlerian schools in his interpretation of the motivating force behind man's activities. He cannot accept either the sex impulse or the will to power as the whole urge, although he definitely believes that the conscious and subconscious activities of man are purposeful. In other words, he concludes that there is a purpose behind all consciousness. He seeks a "master urge" to explain the purpose of man's different instinctive functionings, but unfortunately, he does not give the definite or specific nature of that master urge.

Gestalt psychology, of which Dr. Wolfgang Köhler is the most prominent exponent, is seeking a "totality" of conscious experience. According to this school, the conscious self is a unity and not a combination or sum total of separate instincts and perceptions. The Gestalt psychologists, however, do not as yet give us a complete explanation of this "total" mind—the conscious, subconscious, and superconscious.

We can safely say that there is a general tendency among modern psychiatrists to think that all conscious and subconscious activities of men's minds function purposively and that they are controlled by a unifying principle. There must be a purpose or a reason for the behavior of a man. On the other hand, those of the behaviorist school claim that man is practically a machine and that consciousness itself is only an illusion. These thinkers criticize not only Freud and Jung for their study of the unconscious state of mind but all who believe in the existence of the consciousness of man, not to speak of the existence of God. To a behaviorist God is only an illusion created by the "laziness of mankind." To quote John B. Watson:

In the larger group God or Jehovah takes the place of the family father. Thus even the modern child from the beginning is confronted by the dicta of medicine men—be they the father, the soothsayer of the village, the God, or Jehovah. Having been brought up in this attitude towards authority, he never questions the concepts imposed upon him.[11]

Behaviorists will tell us to study a man's physical make-up if we would understand his behavior. Of course, the psycho-analysts, as well as the Hindu psychologists, admit that there is a great change in the physical state when there is a change in the mind and vice versa. When the mind is affected, there will be a change in the body. But there are still many questions which the behaviorists have yet to answer adequately or satisfactorily. They cannot fully explain many of the cases of psychosis and neurosis by tracing the causes in the structure of the nerves and nerve centers, although it is true that some of the dementia praecox and other cases are cured by insulin, other drugs, and shock treatment. However, in spite of the physiological experiments of these schools, their conclusions are incomplete, for they do not explain the extra-sensory perceptions and superconscious states of mind.

The mechanistic schools have exaggerated their claims for their view of the mechanical nature of the mind. According

[11] John B. Watson, *Behaviorism* (London: Kegan Paul, 1924), p. 4.

to them, mind is a complex mechanism like a modern lino-type, or some other complicated printing machine, which does all the work of a number of men. But we do not find any real explanation of human behavior under extremely complicated and unknown environments and situations. The mechanical view does not give initiative and dynamic re-sourcefulness to the mechanical mind. In the observation of human behavior we fail to find any purposive ingenuity of the unfathomable mind which can be converted into mere functions of material cells or nerve cells. Mechanistic be-haviorism cannot explain the various higher mental faculties or human functions, such as love and sympathy, not to speak of the higher values and spiritual qualities which operate in elevated stages of human society.

On the other hand, the purposivists or hormic psychol-ogists, like Professor McDougall, want to avoid some of the limitations of behaviorism and functionalism by endowing consciousness with purposive faculties. The driving forces are innate in the mind in the form of instincts and urges. Man strives to overcome difficulties and to be master of the situation. Purposivists can better explain complicated human nature although they also fall short of total understanding of human experiences. The same can be said of Gestaltists.

It should be noted here that great emphasis is given to "action" in most of the schools of psychology in America. We may safely say that the major trend in American psy-chology is in the motor aspect of mind. Professor William James can be regarded as the founder of "action psychology" in this country, although Bain and Darwin were the fore-runners. According to James "all consciousness is motor." Münsterberg and Dewey became the great exponents of the school of thought which emphasized activity, achievement, and conduct. The pragmatism of James was greedily taken up by Dewey and others in the field of psychology. As a result we find that the development of mind is measured by its outer expressions and achievements in the objective sense. The quality of intelligence is determined by the measurement of ability in action. Consequently, the subjective element of mind is ignored. In fact, meditation and inner understanding are generally neglected. Professor Gordon Allport of Harvard University gave a beautiful summary of the specialty of American psychology in his speech as chairman of the Society for Psychological Study of Social Issues. He said: "The genius of American psychology lies in its stress upon action or, in slightly dated terminology, upon the motor phase of reflex arc." Again he said: "We seldom record, for example, an individual's unique and subjective pattern of thought life."[12] This tendency of American psychology is easily understood when we consider the major trends of American life and its outlook. The hedonistic outlook on life naturally affects all spheres of activity in a nation. We shall see later that Hindu psychology has quite a different emphasis, as it flourished in a nation where the subjective elements of mind and unique inner mental states play a great part. In fact, spiritual idealism is the most dominant factor in Hindu national life. In his evaluation of American psychology Professor Allport is most accurate. According to the Hindu psychological schools, the greatest expression of mind lies in its total illumination, which is achieved, as we shall see, by the subjective methods of concentration and meditation and consequent mental integration. The mind must be synthesized in order for a person to achieve real success. Greatness of mind can be judged not by its ability in action but rather by its integration and unification.

Hindu psychologists recognize four states of consciousness. To use the terminology of some of them, one can say that

[12] Gordon W. Allport, "The Psychology of Participation," *The Psychological Review*, LII (May, 1945), 117-31

they believe in the sleeping, dreaming, awakened states, and the superconscious—*susupti, swapna, jagrat,* and *turiya.* The sleeping and dreaming states are included in the subconscious. So, according to Western terminology, this amounts to three states—subconscious, conscious, and superconscious. The study of the superconscious is either ignored or considered pathological by most Western psychologists, although Professor William James studied the manifestations of it in his book, *Varieties of Religious Experiences,*[13] and Dr. Müller-Freienfels gives hints of mental telepathy and other such unusual mental phenomena in his treatment of parapsychology in *Evolution of Modern Psychology.*[14] It is also encouraging to note that Professor Rhine of Duke University has made a careful study of what he calls "extrasensory perceptions" in his book, *New Frontiers of the Mind,*[15] to see if he can reach a scientific explanation of certain mental perceptions that are received independently of the sense organs and nervous system.

Although telepathy and clairvoyance seem to be expressions of extrasensory powers, they are not to be confused with the superconscious state or *samadhi.* In fact, the exercise of these extraordinary powers is considered as an obstacle to the attainment of superconscious realization. This is emphasized in the *Yoga Aphorisms of Patanjali* and the *Teachings of Sri Ramakrishna.* However, Patanjali (the father of Hindu psychology) and others recognize these perceptions and even give the methods by which one can develop them although they discourage the use of them if one would attain to true spirituality. Sometimes telepathy, clairvoyance, and other similar powers are manifested in persons without any

[13] William James, *Varieties of Religious Experiences* (London: Longmans, 1929).
[14] Müller-Freienfels, *Evolution of Modern Psychology*, pp. 469-78.
[15] Joseph Banks Rhine, *New Frontiers of the Mind* (London: Faber, 1937).

conscious effort on their part; sometimes they are manifested in the course of the true practice of *yoga* and the right type of concentration and meditation; but they are powers in the worldly sense, and the real seeker after truth is warned not to let them draw him from his goal. In Hindu psychology and other such systems a thorough study has been made of the various stages of superconscious realization and other extrasensory perceptions through *Raja Yoga* practices as given in the *Yoga Aphorisms of Patanjali*. Certain types of lower extrasensory perceptions are discussed in books on *Hatha Yoga*; but we do not propose to describe *Hatha Yoga*, as it is meant primarily for the control of physical laws.

It is of fundamental importance to note that there are distinct differences between the experimental and inferential methods of the Western psychologists and the subjective and intuitive *yoga* practices (mental science or psychology) of the Hindus.[16] The purely objective method cannot be adequately applied to the study of the mind. The psychologist has to interpret the normal and abnormal outer expressions in order to understand the inner states and urges of the mind. He inevitably colors the interpretations by his preconceived notions. Apart from that, a particular expression may have different causes. There is a popular saying that a fool laughs three times over a joke. He laughs first when he sees others laughing; again he laughs when he understands it; and then he laughs thinking what a fool he was not to understand the joke in the first place. As laughter was created by three different causes, so an external expression can be caused by different inner emotions and urges. Consequently, the interpretive method can hardly give convincing understanding of the inner nature of the mind, as neuroses and psychoses may be created in various persons by different

[16] *Yoga* will be discussed elaborately in Chapter XI, " Methods of Superconscious Experience."

subconscious and conscious urges and mental conditions. Therefore, the Hindus have devoted themselves thoroughly to the subjective methods of psychology which give a clear and conclusive understanding of the total mind.

Western thinkers may be inclined to question the validity of psychological study in India, as they may find that Hindu psychology is not experimental in the sense of the Western schools of experimental psychology. Nevertheless, it can never be said that Hindu psychology is not empirical, for it is based on the study of the experience of the mind. Brentano and a number of others of his school did not ascribe much value to modern experimental psychology, although empirical psychology was considered by them to be extremely valuable because they were interested in the nature of the mind. Professor Boring evidently does not esteem Brentano highly as a psychologist, as he considers him and his followers to be philosophers whose major interest was in the understanding of the whole.[17] Such historians and others may find it difficult to appreciate the contributions of Hindu psychology, and they may dismiss the whole system as a philosophical treatise or as mystical literature. It would be unfair to come to such a conclusion, as Hindu psychology gives definite methods not only for knowing the nature of the mind but also for developing its powers. Occidental psychological methods are not the only way of knowing the mind.

We should clearly understand what is meant by the subjective and intuitive method of Hindu psychology. It does not mean philosophizing about the nature of the mind or having a conceptual knowledge thereof, but rather training the total mind of the individual, including thought, emotion, and will. It does not depend on the interpretive

---

[17] Edwin G. Boring, *A History of Experimental Psychology* (London: Appleton, 1929), p. 349.

method, as interpretation of the outer expressions of the mind may not always be reliable. Hindu psychologists firmly believe that psychological facts and development can be verified and developed through personal mental growth. A sincere follower of the methods of psychological development can achieve unique growth and can verify the principles discovered through the experiences of many persons. As they believe in the verifiability of different mental experiences, Hindu psychologists, although subjective and intuitive, are scientific as well as practical and dynamic.

Psychology in the West is now regarded as dynamic by many outstanding psychologists. It is our opinion that Hindu psychology is more dynamic, as it trains the individual mind to manifest all its latent powers. We will see in the chapters on "Meditation" and "Methods of Superconscious Experience" that through systematic psychological practices the dynamic powers of mind evolve and make an individual mind powerful enough to be of service to others in integrating their emotions and other mental processes.

Hindu psychologists are primarily interested in the study and development of the total mind rather than in the different functions considered separately. The experimental psychologists of the West are interested in the particular phases of mental activity. Some of them go to an extreme in their specialization when they study only nerve reactions and think that they will be able to comprehend the mind itself while they study merely the instruments of the mind. It is interesting to note what Professor Hocking rightly says in his evaluation of Western psychology: "But the extant science or sciences of mind have presented us not the mind itself, but substitutes for mind, . . .—Near-minds, we may call them."[18]

[18] W. E. Hocking, " Mind and Near Mind," *Proceedings of the Sixth International Congress of Philosophy*. ed. Edgar Sheffield Brightman (London: Longmans, 1927), p. 203.

And again he says: "The several Near-minds of the scientific psychology have their worth and their actuality; but they have life only as organs of mind."[19] It will not be out of place to remember here that Hindus accept the existence of mind apart from and independent of the nerves. Brentano and the Gestaltists are no doubt interested to a great extent in the total experience of the mind, but they do not seem to go far enough to cover the whole range of mental experiences, as we have said already, for they never consider the superconscious. The psychologists of the unconscious—Freud, Adler, Jung, and others—also fall short, as we have seen. We make bold to say that the Western psychologists are mostly concerned with the different phases of mental functioning by taking them separately and individually in their experimental methods, while Hindu psychologists are primarily interested in the study of the total mind, as they feel that the different functions—consciousness, unconsciousness, superconsciousness, cognition, volition, and conation—cannot be really separated. Moreover, they are interrelated. As we know, any thought creates an emotional reaction resulting in activity. A thought or a concept creates an emotion within, such as attraction or repulsion, pleasure or displeasure, love or hatred. We are also aware of our emotions; as such, thought and emotion cannot be isolated and observed separately. Emotional urges make the mind active. It is almost impossible to observe activity of the mind (function of will) as separate from either thought or emotion. Nor can we observe a thought as separate from emotion or activity of the mind. Neither can emotions be isolated from the knowledge content of the mind and its dynamic expression, however subtle they may be. Thought, emotion, and will are inseparably connected. That is the reason Hindu psychologists study these functions together when they try to develop and

[19] *Ibid.*, p. 215.

integrate the mind. Then again, they consider that the fullest development of mind can be achieved only when it reaches the superconscious. A student of psychology also has knowledge of the contents of the unconscious (*samaskaras*) in the process of the development of the superconscious. In fact, a study of the unconscious when isolated from conscious training of the mind is extremely unsafe, as we shall discuss in the chapter on the Subconscious Mind. So according to Hindu psychologists, one cannot really study and know one state of mind properly without total integration of the mind.

Most of the American psychologists seem to give extreme emphasis to the motor aspect of the mind. In other words, their chief interest is to know the activity, the motor consequences of mental life, in order to find out how the mind acts and reacts from the motor point of view. On the other hand, Hindu psychologists try to understand and strengthen the whole mind. Therefore, they are especially interested in the development of character and personality, which can be achieved only by integration of the mind. We appreciate some of the Western psychologists like Professor Allport and Professor Allers who are interested in the total personality of man.[20]

It should be mentioned that we do not minimize the importance of a great number of psychologists in India who taught psychological principles before the time of Patanjali (about 150 B.C.). Applied psychology was taught in the *Upanishads*, the *Bhagavad-Gita*, and the *Sankhya* system. The Buddhists also gave many definite and practical ideas of applied psychology for the unification and strengthening of the mind, as well as definite instructions for the total enlightenment of the mind. In fact, Patanjali gives a syste-

[20] Gordon W. Allport, *Personality, A Psychological Interpretation* (London: Constable, 1937); and Rudolph Allers, *The Psychology of Character* (New York: Sheed & Ward, 1943).

matic treatise on *yoga,* though many of his concepts are based on Sankhya thought.

Hindus have developed their psychology mainly in the course of religious unfoldment. The Western psychoanalysts —Charcot, Janêt, Freud, Adler, Jung, and others—began their research in the abnormal states of the mind. The physiological psychologists are more interested in the study of the nerve reactions and functionings of the nervous system than in the mind itself. Professor Hocking of Harvard University aptly calls this a study of the "near-mind." It should be remembered that it is extremely unsafe, to say the least, to generalize the findings from the study of the abnormal mind and apply them to fairly normal minds. Freud and others make superficial remarks about the religious tendencies of man in terms of sex, and they try to find the "death" or "destructive" tendencies even in normal and supernormal minds. Actually, the supernormal minds function in a manner quite different from normal and abnormal cases. This is the reason that the unfortunate generalizations of many of the psychotherapeutists regarding spiritual experiences are extremely inaccurate and unscientific. They are far from the truth.

The science of psychology was developed mainly by the Hindus as they studied the methods by which they reached the highest religious experience—the superconscious state or *samadhi.* It is the only method of understanding and controlling the mind in order that a higher consciousness may be reached. According to the *Yoga Aphorisms of Patanjali,* the mind becomes thoroughly illumined and can transcend even the limitation of the nervous system when it is controlled and unified in the course of concentration and deep meditation. The mind can immediately and directly reach another plane, the superconscious state, in which it experiences reality. This is explained by Swami Vivekananda in *Raja Yoga*:

There is a still higher plane upon which the mind can work. It can go beyond consciousness. Just as unconscious work is beneath consciousness, so there is another work which is above consciousness, and which is not accompanied with the feeling of egoism. The feeling of egoism is only on the middle plane. . . . By the effects, by the results of the work, we know that which is below, and that which is above. When a man goes into deep sleep he enters a plane beneath consciousness. He works the body all the time, he breathes, he moves the body, perhaps, in his sleep, without any accompanying feeling of ego; he is unconscious, and when he returns from his sleep he is the same man who went into it. The sum total of the knowledge which he had before he went into the sleep remains the same; it does not increase at all. No enlightenment does come. But when a man goes into *samadhi*, if he goes into it a fool, he comes out a sage.[21]

Religious ideals and expressions are essential to the fulfillment and culmination of consciousness in this supersensuous state. To Hindus, religion is not a barrier to psychological development and understanding; it is the very basis for the total illumination of the mind.

According to Hindu psychologists, when the mind is subjected to the discipline of *yoga* practices the fine nerve tissues of the body undergo a consequent transformation. The physical and mental forces of man are refined and unified, resulting in emotional balance, development of adamantine will, and physical poise. A man who has experienced *samadhi* or superconscious realization understands the whole mind—conscious, subconscious, and superconscious. He also reaches a stage where the mind functions independently of the nervous system, as seen in the teachings of Swami Brahmananda.

---

[21] *The Complete Works of Swami Vivekananda* (Mayavati, Almora, Himalayas: Advaita Ashrama, 1931), I, 180. Hereafter, this source of reference will be referred to as *Works*.

In fact, to him the whole mind appears like a mirror in which he can see the truth revealed. Again, this unified mind that has been subjected to discipline through the practices of concentration, meditation, and other processes, becomes a center of power. When a man is master of his own mental forces, he will be able to understand and influence the minds of others. He is well established in poise and creates an atmosphere of peace. When anyone enters the presence of such a person, he consciously or unconsciously absorbs the peaceful atmosphere and derives poise and benefit from the contact. A man of superconscious realization can be compared to a luminous substance which radiates light. It not only illumines itself but also objects within its radius. Similarly, a man with a unified mind emanates wisdom and strength to others.

CHAPTER II

Cognition

IT IS only within the last fifty years that the people of the Western world have come to realize the importance of psychology and see that it is not merely a philosophical or speculative study but also an indispensable factor in adjustment to the demands of practical everyday life. Hindus, on the contrary, have been aware of this for centuries. For hundreds of years they have been using psychology not only as a method for the unfoldment of religious truth, the basis of their deep philosophy, but also as an aid in the field of medicine and the key to health, poise, and harmonious living.

Generally speaking, it is the more utilitarian aspects of psychology that have had a popular appeal in the West, especially in America—for various reasons. In the field of medicine, for instance, more and more attention is being given to the study of the effect of the mind upon the nervous system, especially in cases of so-called "functional" ailments. Physicians now say that the harmful effects of unbalanced mental or emotional states upon physical well-being cannot be overestimated, and they are emphasizing the need of mental and emotional control as essential to good health. Medicines, drugs, and even surgery have been known to fail in cases where the patient did not have control of his mind or lacked emotional stability.

Again, a knowledge of psychology is proving to be very useful in the business world. Those with commercial interests, especially in the field of advertising, have made a careful study of the power of suggestion in order to increase their sales. Enormous sums of money are being spent to influence buyers, not only in display but also in the use of radio, and every conceivable device is employed to interest the public in the products that are being advertised. In many businesses, courses in psychology are given to the sales clerks so that they may be more successful in dealing with customers. For instance, they are taught to give more attention to a man who is shopping, as he is likely to buy what he wants in the first store to which he goes, while a woman prefers to "shop around" and compare values. Thus it is evident that influencing the minds of others has come to be of great importance even in the business world.

Then there are people who want charm, beauty, or a magnetic personality. Some desire to be successful politically, to gain control over others, or to develop strong will power. All these and similar wants have created a large market for books on psychology of a pleasant popular variety, some of which are of little value. They reflect the need of more and more help for the people in mastering their problems, however, and they also show that the public is beginning to appreciate the understanding of the mind as a guide to practical living.

Finally, there are those who want to understand psychology for its own sake. Almost everyone, at some time or other, has experienced a desire to know more about himself. "Who am I?" "Why do I exist?" and "What is my relationship to this objective world that I face every day?" are only a few of the questions that cannot fail to present themselves to an inquiring and intelligent mind. Yes, "Know thyself" is still the key to wisdom, as it was in the days of Socrates; and this self-knowledge as developed in Hindu psychology is the way to freedom, truth, and harmonious living.

The study of psychology is essentially a study of the mind, its functionings, its reactions to the objective world, and the methods by which it obtains knowledge. For convenience we can define the mind as "that which classifies, judges, and co-ordinates the impressions and sensations gathered from the outside world—that which knows and knows that it knows."[1] This, of course, brings us face to face with several problems. For instance, who is the knower and what is the nature of knowledge? How do I know that I know, and how can I be sure that my knowledge is correct? Does the mind have a separate existence apart from physical brain matter, or is it only a bundle of sensations—the product of the sense organs and the nervous system? We shall deal with each of these questions in the course of this study, beginning with cognition or knowledge.

It has been shown by the great physicist and botanist, Sir J. C. Bose of Calcutta, India, that even plants and the simplest organisms have certain sensations and reactions that, of course, become more pronounced in the higher forms of life. The lower animals are provided with sense organs through which they gather a specialized and peculiar knowledge of external things. Dogs, for instance, depend a great deal upon their keen sense of smell; even a serpent knows something of the world about him through his reaction to sound, although he does not have the usual outer organs for hearing. In studying reptiles, the Western psychologists have found that while "some (lizards) apparently have auditory sensitivity; others (snakes) apparently do not."[2] Animals have an instinctive knowledge that is very accurate, though limited in scope as compared with cognition and awareness in man.

There was a school of thinkers in India called *Charbakas*

[1] Sri Sankaracharya, *Vivekachudamani*, pp. 93-94.
[2] N. R. F. Maier and T. C. Schneirla, *Principles of Animal Psychology* (New York: McGraw-Hill Book Co., Inc., 1935), p. 219.

who, like the behaviorists and other psychologists of similar
type in the West, declared that thought processes, cognition,
and emotion are merely the products of nerve reaction, that
the so-called "mind" is only a bundle of successive sensations
dependent upon the nervous system and physical brain
matter. Consciousness has no independent existence. According to Watson:

> It [consciousness] is a plain assumption just as unprovable, just
> as unapproachable, as the old concept of the Soul. And to the
> behaviorist the two terms are essentially identical, so far as con-
> cerns their metaphysical implications. . . . They do not tell us
> what consciousness is, but merely begin to put things into it by
> assumption; and then when they come to analyze consciousness,
> naturally they find in it just what they put into it.[3]

Watson and others assume that the existence of the entity
depends on the possibility of objective observation. The behaviorists seem to forget that they cannot observe objectively
their own thinking processes, yet they believe that they can
evaluate the psychological concepts of Wundt, James, and
others. They also assume that they have something with
which "to observe behavior." As Watson says:

> Why don't we make what we can observe the real field of
> psychology? Let us limit ourselves to things that can be observed,
> and formulate laws concerning only those things. Now what can
> we observe? Well, we can observe behavior and what the organism
> does and says.[4]

The interest of the behaviorists is to observe behavior "in
terms of stimulus and response."

If we examine these statements closely, we will see that
these psychologists are confusing consciousness with sensa-

[3] John B. Watson, *Behaviorism* (2nd ed.; New York: W. W. Norton & Co.,
Inc., 1930) p. 5.
[4] *Ibid.*, p. 6.

tions, and the senses (the instruments for obtaining knowledge) with thought and emotion. A simple illustration will explain this. Electricity acts through wires and a bulb to produce light, but the electricity is neither the wires nor the bulb; the light is the result of its action. Electricity cannot be seen or described except in terms of its effect. We can only prove its existence through the use of an external medium. Similarly, the mind acts in ordinary persons through the brain and nervous system (as mentioned in Chapter I), and it can only be understood and interpreted by the way it uses the powers at its disposal. Again, if the mind were only the product of nerve stimuli it could be observed objectively. But the observation of the mind and thought current of an individual is not objectively possible and cannot be done successfully without subjective insight. How do you know what your friends are thinking? How can anyone know exactly what is going on in the mind of another? A man may appear to be listening to a sermon, but in reality his mind is busily occupied elsewhere—at home, at the bank, or thinking of some private worry. Yet, to an objective observer, he seems to be giving attention to the speaker. He alone knows what is really going on in his mind.

Another fact that the physiological, behaviorist, and mechanical psychologists seem to have overlooked is the absolute necessity for permanence and integration in the mind of the observer, so that he may be able to classify and co-ordinate the impressions and experiences gained through his objective study. If his mind is only a bundle of successive sensations, how can he possibly hold the memory of more than one sensation at a time? Again, how can one sensation, which he himself is at the moment, be the observer of another sensation which is the object of his study? In other words, if I am nothing but a collection of sensations, how can that "I" become the observer of "you" who are nothing but another conglomeration of sensations? How can "I" correlate this information if "I" can be conscious of only one thing, followed immediately by something else? Obviously, there must be some permanent factor that holds together these impressions and differentiates between them. This brings us to the conclusion that it must be the mind that perceives, experiences, and consequently becomes a knower of the objective world. We should also remember that the successive sensations cannot give us a total picture of a thing unless there is a background as the receptacle of these sensations. For instance, the moving pictures cannot become perceptible unless there is a permanent background on which the constant moving pictures are impressed.

Besides, the behaviorists, with their conception of sensation as the mind itself, cannot explain the fact of memory. They do not tell us how and where the different sensations are preserved in the form of memory. We are compelled to accept that there is a permanent receptacle of the residuals of experiences which is the mind.

And we do not only have the cognition of the objective and perceived world; we also have the cognition of the internal awareness. Pleasurable and painful mental conditions are also cognized by ourselves. These pleasurable and painful past and present mental states and also the apprehensions and anxieties of the future are cognized by human beings. Such experiences could not be interpreted as mere successive sensations or nerve reactions. There must be something which is in the background of this cognition of the mental states themselves.

We all are aware of inner emotions. The emotions may be either a reaction to external perception or they may be inner urges. We perceive our own feelings of love, affection, hatred, envy, fear, anxiety, and worry. If there is no separate existence of mind apart from mere succession of sensations, then the perception of our inner emotions would not be possible. We cannot perceive previously experienced facts and their inner emotional reactions if we do not have something to preserve them in the form of memories. In fact, memory itself becomes impossible if there is no receptacle of successive sensations. In order to understand these facts we can refer to the previous example of moving pictures. It is the experience of every thinking man that he is aware of his own emotions. It will not be out of place to note also that we all have a kind of consciousness of our persistent awareness of ourselves. As philosopher Descartes says: "I think, so I exist." One cannot explain the different states and processes of mind without the acceptance of a permanent mind.

Having established the necessity for the existence of the mind[5] which is independent of mere sensations, we shall consider the ways in which it functions with regard to perception of the objective world. How does the knower gain knowledge? Who is the knower? What is the relationship of the mind to external things?

According to Western psychologists, the sense organs receive stimuli that are passed on by the nervous system to the brain cells. Even the psychologists who accept the theory of independent existence of the mind regard it as passive, while the objective world is conceived as dynamic, impressing itself upon the mind through the nervous system. However, they do not tell us how continuous and successive sensations, received from the same object, are unified in the mind that is passive. The Charles River flows in a continuous stream; yet this successive flow of water, which is the Charles River, gives the appearance of unity and oneness because of its bed. Similarly, regardless of how quick the successive sensations

---

[5] *Antahkarana,* or internal instrument, according to *Brahmasutra,* Vedanta Aphorism.

may be, it would not be possible to get a complete picture of
a thing without a permanent entity of mind.

Gestalt psychologists in their interpretation of the total
mind are nearing an understanding of it. They conceive that
the entire object is impressed on the whole mind. Some of the
"action" psychologists, and a few others, try to eliminate this
problem of unification of sensations in a passive mind by
conceding that the mind becomes active when stimulated
by impressions, but the majority seems to think that the
mind is perfectly passive. Difficulties arise here because successive and individual sensations could not possibly become
integrated in a passive mind, either by themselves or by the
mind as a passive receptacle. James, Münsterberg, and others
of actionist psychology, do not eliminate the difficulty in
their psychomotor ideas, as they say that stimuli are trans-
posed into responses. Mind seems to be entirely dependent
on the stimuli even though they measure the mind by its
ability in action. Gestalt and action psychologists also seem
to fail to endow mind with independence of sense stimuli, and
so they limit the scope of the mind. Even those psychologists
who concede that the mind may become active when external
sensations are received fail to explain how these fragmentary
impressions can become unified. Some psychologists say that
the mind cannot really know an object but can know only
the sensations of that object. In that case, we could not know
anything of the objective world except the sensations thereof.
This would also mean that our knowledge would be inaccurate, as we have to depend upon sensations which constantly vary according to the nature and conditions of the
perceiving person, who is also an aggregate of successive and
changeable sensations. We often observe that a particular
sensation of an object is interpreted by different observers in
different ways according to the predisposition of the observ-

ing minds. Besides, the perceiving mind also will change, as it is supposed to be in a flux.

According to Indian psychologists, it is the mind that reaches out to the objective world through the sense organs and nervous system, drawing its sensations and impressions through them and unifying the experiences gathered into coherent information or knowledge. The word "mind" corresponds to the Vedantic word *antahkarana* (inner instrument)[6] which has four functions: (1) *manas*, the oscillating or indecisive faculty of mind; (2) *buddhi*, the decisive state which determines that "this is a tree and not a man"; (3) *ahamkara*, the state which ascertains that "I know"; (4) *chitta*, the storehouse of mental states which makes remembrance and reference possible. We can call this the "mind-stuff."[7] According to the Hindu system of thought (Vedanta), *antahkarana* stands between the Self and the object and receives the object of perception, assuming its form as a whole. Gestalt psychology of the West has a similar conception, although there is some difference. *Antahkarana* is the inner instrument through which the subject knows the object by identification. It is not the Self. Self is consciousness and not the product of the relationship between subject and object. It is the underlying, self-illumining principle. Self, or *Atma*, is called *Sakshi*, the unchangeable Reality. It remains only as the witness. Mind, or *antahkarana*, gets its power by association with the Self, or *Atma*, which is the same as *Brahman*, or the Absolute. It has become seemingly individualized by virtually limiting itself by ignorance.[8] We do not propose to discuss further the metaphysical side of the problem. It has been mentioned to complete the Hindu idea of perception and its different aspects.

---

[6] *Vivarana Prameya Samgraha* and *Vedanta Paribhasa*.

[7] The *Sankhya* system of thought in India offers a great deal of material on the different functionings of the "mind-stuff."

[8] *Works*, I, 200-201.

c*

There is a difference between the Greek conception of the soul and its functions and the Hindu conception of *Atma* and its functions. Greek psychologists, including Aristotle, conceive activity in the soul itself, although there are differences among various Greek thinkers as to the nature of the activity. But *Atma* of the Hindus is the unchangeable Reality, the Great Witness, Consciousness Itself, *Sakshi Chaitanya.*

Hindu psychologists conceive the internal implement for perception as the *indriya* (sense),[9] which is independent of the outer sense organs and nervous system, although it operates through them. The *indriya* is not the mind, though the mind uses it as an implement.[10] A definite difference between the two is shown in the following:

> Know that the Soul, who sits within, is the master of the chariot, and the body the chariot. Consider the intellect [*buddhi*] as the charioteer, and the mind [*manas*] the reins. The senses [*indriyas*] are the horses and their roads are the sense objects.[11]

The *indriya* is not passive; it is dynamic. It functions actively to reach out to the objective world and stimulate the nervous system and sense organs.[12] The conception of *indriya* is utterly foreign to Western psychologists, and there will be considerable doubt among them concerning its existence. However, as we study perception we shall see that the Hindus have good reason to conceive the mind as actively seeking sensation, and that the existence of *indriya* is logical.

Almost all the psychologists of the East and West accept perception as the most direct method of obtaining knowledge. I see you; therefore, I believe that you exist. If I also

[9] *Vivarana Prameya Samgraha* and *Vedanta Paribhasa. Indriya* is translated as "sense" as there is no other appropriate word for it. Some may consider this an unusual use of the word "sense."

[10] *Katha Upanishad* 3:3.

[11] *Ibid.,* 3:3 and 4.

[12] This is further elaborated in *Vedanta Paribhasa.*

touch you I am convinced that you are there. But suppose you are passing me on the street and I do not see you. I may be looking in your direction; my eyes are still functioning and your image is reflected upon the retina; yet I do not know that you are there. Why? If my mind were passive, I could not avoid seeing you. The stimulation to my mind from the optic nerve would have informed me, but obviously some part of the mind was not reacting to the stimuli. The mind was not reaching out to the external world and stimulating the *indriya* to observe; consequently, I could pass you without knowing that you were there. This also explains so-called "absent-mindedness," where the internal instruments of perception, the *indriya* and the mind, were not concerning themselves with the objective world and I became forgetful of external matters. The *indriya* was preoccupied or busily engaged with something else.

Although serpents have no external organs of hearing, they have some internal means to cognize the sound. The Indian conception of *indriya* explains this peculiar perceptive quality of serpents. Plants also seem to have no external organs; yet, as Sir J. C. Bose demonstrated, they have certain types of sensation. This proves that they have some internal instrument of sensation.

Extrasensory perceptions cannot be explained if we do not accept this inner sense of the mind. This will be treated more fully in another chapter. It is enough to say here that the so-called extrasensory perceptions take place without the least contact between the sense organs and the object perceived. Here the *indriya* is gathering experiences by projecting itself independently of the nervous system and the sense organs. The knowledge thus obtained, without direct contact with the object, can be tested to determine its validity as true knowledge. Visions (not hallucinations) and similar experiences are well-known examples of perception of this type. In dreams, or in certain extraordinary states, some persons have had perceptions that were proved to be prophetic. All this indicates the *indriya's* independence of the sense organs and nervous system.

There is another aspect of perception that needs to be considered. This is the power of the mind to interpret the sensations of external objects or sense stimuli. According to Western psychology, when an object is perceived, its image is reflected by light waves upon the retina of the eye in an inverted form, and from this image the mind draws its conclusions about the object. It not only determines size, color, proportion, and the various properties of the object, but also sees it in its relation to other things of like or opposite nature. The eye alone could not do all this. It is the mind that correlates and unifies this information. The question will arise: How do we know that the knowledge received corresponds to the reality of the object? On a dark night a trunk of a tree may appear to be a robber, a friend, or a ghost, depending upon the mental state of the person who sees it. It is the internal instrument of perception that differentiates between these impressions, classifying them as true or false and choosing the one that seems to be most accurate. By comparison with former experiences the mind "recognizes" that the dark object in question is neither a man nor a ghost but is only the trunk of a tree. Similarly, the mind discriminates between the evidence produced by the senses to obtain knowledge of the external world, the universe, and of other minds.

Although direct perception is generally conceded as the most convincing proof of knowledge, there are other methods also that may be accepted as valid, especially in cases where direct and immediate perception would be impossible. For instance, we accept knowledge upon authority. How do we know that there is war in the world? We cannot perceive it directly. We are obliged to rely upon the testimony of others, upon newspapers, and the information gathered by people who are witnessing it in order to know that a conflict is raging. It would be folly to say that there cannot be a war because we cannot experience it directly. When the sources of information can be checked as reliable and trustworthy, whether it is a question of an event of history or the effects of a poison, the conclusions reached may be accepted as true even though they have been proved or experienced by others.

Another method of obtaining knowledge is by inference. It has been observed that when a fire burns it produces smoke. Consequently, if we see smoke we infer that there must be a fire somewhere that is causing it. If volumes of smoke are pouring out of a building, we do not wait to see flames before notifying the fire department. We know by inference that a fire is there and that it will destroy the building if it is not put out.

Inference and authority are not the same, although some people try to classify them together. Authority can stand alone, independent of inference. For example, the great fire of Chicago was a fact that can be accepted upon authority. But we cannot infer it now since the direct evidence of the destruction must have been cleared away long ago.

Just as the sources of authoritative knowledge must be scrutinized for reliability, so also does the proof of inferential knowledge depend upon the validity of its conclusions and the major and minor terms. Great care should be taken in establishing these; otherwise, the inferential knowledge will be misleading or actually false. For that matter, direct perceptions have to be scrutinized also, as the subjective element in every factor in perception contributes a great deal. In fact, perceptions vary according to the interpretations that are given in the light of the notions of the mind. Western philosophers, as well as Indian philosophers, mostly agree in recognizing the contributions of the mind. Professor Eddington, in *The Philosophy of Physical Science*, logically and factually tries to prove that even scientific knowledge, which is supposed to be authentic, seems to be relative, because he, too, believes that there is a subjective element even in scientific perceptions.[13] We can again cite the celebrated illustration of Vedantic epistemology. On a dark night when a man looks at a trunk of a tree, he often conceives it as a thief, or a friend, or a policeman, according to the preconceived notions that he has. Scrutiny is therefore needed in all these forms of cognition and knowledge.

Induction and deduction are the methods of inference, and they are used by modern scientists. In the deductive method a general statement is taken and from that is deduced a particular truth. The inductive method is just the opposite; scientific facts are used to aim at a general conclusion. Almost all scientists directly or indirectly use inferential methods as a means of cognition.

Indian Vedantic epistemology and psychology also accept comparison, postulation, and nonperception as the means of new knowledge. We are not discussing these points, as they are not vitally related to the science of psychology. They are studied in epistemology.

The question to which we referred in the earlier pages regarding the validity of knowledge needs a little mention here. As this is also vitally connected with epistemology, we should not elaborately discuss the true criterion of knowledge or cognition. No philosopher or psychologist can help questioning the validity of knowledge. Consequently, a few propositions of the Indian schools of thought should be briefly stated. Some thinkers, such as the pragmatists of America, regard knowledge as a fact of true cognition when it has practical value; the standards of real knowledge depend on its

[13] A. S. Eddington, *Philosophy of Physical Science* (Cambridge University Press, 1929).

practical application in life. We can accept a hypothesis and work out certain schemes which may have practical value. Yet the hypothesis may not be true, as it will be contradicted by the later discovery and perception. For instance, the astronomical theory of solar rotation was later contradicted by the discovery of earthly rotation; yet, for many practical purposes, the astronomical calculations of the previous generations were useful.

There are some among Indians, as well as among Western realistic thinkers, who hold that cognition is true when it corresponds to real fact. This needs clarification regarding the very conception of "real." When we are living on a certain plane of existence things may seem to be real, yet when we are transported to other planes of existence those very things may be unreal. When a person with jaundice looks at certain objects they appear to be yellow. So long as the jaundiced condition remains, the perceptions will be colored by it. Racial discrimination and differentiation are often based on opinions and prejudices of those who are on the same plane of existence or who have similar ideas and interests. Although the opinions and prejudices may not actually be based on facts, they are regarded as "real" and consequently the same patterns of understanding and behavior are followed by other persons. When a man dreams, the dream experiences are also real so long as the dream state remains.

There is also another viewpoint among both Indian and Western thinkers that knowledge or cognition must be coherent to the other experiences. It must be in harmony with other states of life and experiences. This view can also be questioned according to the arguments against the previous viewpoint, namely, the correspondence theory of knowledge. The Vedantic test of knowledge is that it must never be contradicted at any time, and knowledge or true cognition must consist in its noncontradiction and newness.

Hallucinations, dreams, and the ordinary perceptions of the awakened state have certain cognitive value, yet hallucinations and dreams vanish when our awakened cognitive state becomes operative. Similarly, when a man rises to the superconscious state (*samadhi*), or the fourth state of consciousness which will be described in one of the later chapters, the awakened experiences, that is to say, our ordinary sense perceptions and other such experiences, are contradicted. This does not mean that Indian philosophy regards the awakened cognitions as hallucinations. It only means that the awakened cognitions are of relative types, such as Professor Eddington describes in *The Philosophy of Physical Science*. The only ultimate, uncontradicted, and unitary knowledge is the knowledge one has at the time of spiritual realization (*samadhi*). This whole evaluation of the different types of cognition comes within the scope of epistemology proper. It requires, no doubt, considerable discussion in a separate book. Yet in psychology proper one should understand the criterion of true cognition.

The mental functionings in the form of cognition have considerable influence over the body, as we shall discuss in the following chapter on emotion. The mental states and processes, whether or not they are in the form of cognition, emotion, or volition, have tremendous influence on the mind itself and also on the body. Although these three functionings are correlated, they are studied separately for the sake of clarity and understanding.

CHAPTER III

Emotion

IN OUR previous discussion of the processes of cognition or knowledge it was mentioned that every act of cognition has a response within the mind. At the same time, knowledge is inseparably connected with an inner emotional reaction; we cannot separate knowledge from its emotional content. It is the purpose of this discussion to present the factors inherent in the human mind which condition man's reaction to his surroundings, and we shall consider how these factors can become constructive elements in a person's adjustment to his environment and can contribute to his happiness.

In addition to cognition we have primitive urges or impulses. Man not only has emotional experiences resulting from external sensations but he also has primitive urges independent of any sensation or perception. Some Western psychologists, such as Professor William James and C. G. Lange, have concluded that emotions generally have their origin in sensations or perceptions. They also admit the existence of primitive instinctive urges.

First, let us understand all the emotional reactions of the human mind. Our interest in the understanding of emotions is not theoretical, as it is of vital importance in human life and human conduct. A man's conduct cannot be understood unless we comprehend the inner springs of his actions. These inner springs are what the great psychologists call the instinctive urges or primitive impulses. They are the driving forces of man's life and activity. Therefore, we want to know not only our own driving forces but also those that govern the conduct of other individuals.

The interest in the study of emotions is of practical value. Moreover, we realize that a man's normal life cannot be well established unless he has proper understanding and proper use of his various emotions. Let us review briefly the five primitive urges or emotions present in all human beings.[1] It may seem that we are arbitrarily classifying the emotions. It is recognized, however, that they are interrelated within themselves and with other emotions; yet for the sake of concrete understanding of our emotional life we are mentioning five specific urges: (1) We observe that there is an inherent impulse in people known as self-preservation. It is, no doubt, of primary importance yet it produces many secondary emotions or what we may call prospective and retrospective emotions, namely: apprehension, anxiety, fear, and such other responses. Every animal has an abundance of this emotion of self-preservation. Even the child shows this instinct before it begins to know anything about itself or its environment. (2) Then there is the urge of self-expression to be considered. We not only struggle to live and prolong our lives, but we also want to express ourselves. If we do not have proper avenues of self-expression, we become miserable. We also find that if this particular urge is extremely accentuated it creates considerable disturbance in our lives. Self-expression is associated with a number of other urges, such as aggression and submission. (3) The sex impulse becomes a strong force

[1] The emotions are differently classified by various outstanding thinkers. It is interesting to note that William I. Thomas and Florian Znaniecki mention four wishes of man: (1) new experience, (2) security, (3) response, and (4) recognition. See William I. Thomas and Florian Znaniecki, *The Polish Peasant in Europe and America*, Vol. III, *Life Record of an Immigrant* (Boston: Richard G. Badger, The Gorham Press, 1919), especially pp. 33 and 57.

in motivating different activities in all beings. We not only want to express ourselves but we want to perpetuate our existence in the form of our children and reproduce the race so that it may continue. There is a pleasure element in the very expression of this impulse. This urge is associated with love, sympathy, affection, envy, jealousy, and many other secondary prospective as well as retrospective emotions. (4) As a result of the gregarious urge or desire for companionship, human beings find it difficult to live alone; they want company. When they cannot express themselves or their emotions of love, affection, or sympathy, they feel suffocated. Many persons feel extremely alone when they have no outlet for their emotions. Some thinkers are of the opinion that man seeks company for self-preservation so that he can fight the battle for life and have different types of pleasure with his fellow beings. According to them, this urge is a phase of self-preservation. We do not agree with such interpretations. When we deeply study human beings, we find that the gregarious instinct is an independent urge. The accompanying secondary emotions are love, envy, jealousy, and other such responses. (5) With the impulse of knowledge, man wants to know not only himself and all the desires within him but also about his environment, other people, and nature. It is not that we acquired this urge as we began to develop our civilization, but it is an inherent quality of mind. This urge of knowledge also has secondary emotions. We have already discussed, in the previous chapter, that the element of knowledge is present in various forms not only in man, civilized and uncivilized, but also in animals.

All these five primitive urges are component urges and they do not always work independently and separately. They are often linked with other emotions. Take, for instance, a primitive urge of self-preservation which is associated with fear and anxiety. We do not know how many persons have a

peculiar complex of fear of ghosts. It sounds amusing, but
let us give an example. We know that this so-called ridiculous
emotion of fear of ghosts will create many other different
emotions. Most people have heard about ghosts and have
certain notions about them. When one goes to an empty
dark house, particularly after any recent misfortune of death,
one feels rather uncomfortable and nervous. If a few squeaks
are heard when the door is opened, the person at once jumps
to the conclusion that someone is walking around inside,
and the first impulse is to run away from the place. We know
of occasions when people actually tried to run away, and it
was not in India but right here in American cities. We
happen to know personally of one occasion when some people
were frightened. On inquiry it was found that the floors
were cracking owing to their construction and the expansion
caused by heat. When the people realized that it was not a
ghost but only the heat that was making the cracking sounds,
the result was laughter, or the emotion of amusement, when
they understood how foolish they had been to think that
there was a ghost in that particular house.

We have fear, then curiosity, and finally amusement successively occurring in many of our experiences. It is difficult
to separate these primitive urges from the secondary emotions; they are, as it were, linked together. All the primitive
urges are associated with other emotions such as fear, amusement, laughter, anxiety, apprehension, and remorse. Some
times, we are likely to become apprehensive of the presence
of these primary and secondary emotions and urges within
us. Being worried, we create certain disorders in our minds;
our behavior is changed, and our conduct becomes re-
morseful. We ask ourselves why we had these apprehensions, worries, and anxieties. We know that because of them
we often wreck our nervous systems. Then we become re-
morseful and regret that we have indulged ourselves in such

expressions of emotion which have ruined our health. If we control ourselves, we are amused that we were so foolish as to have ruined ourselves; we should have known better. In this way the emotions act and react, creating many by-products in the form of functional ailments and disturbances. When these primitive emotions lose their proper balance and create many strong secondary emotions, they cause conflicts in our lives.

We have higher ideas and evaluate ourselves as to what we should or should not do. When we become a little emotional, we think that it is not right to be so. Let us take jealousy, for instance. We are extremely fond of a person. Then someone else comes to like him, and we become jealous. We cannot help relating one thing we have observed in this country, and we hope you will not be offended. It seems that people have formed particular notions that an individual can like or love only one person. Sometimes they ask: "Can a religious teacher have more than one student?" It seems to an Oriental a shocking question, and we think that it would be shocking to an American professor if any student asked: "Sir, can you have more than one pupil?" We believe any teacher or professor would be extremely offended if he were challenged in that way.

Unfortunately, we find that many people in the pseudo-religious organizations seem to think that teachers can have only one student. The others become extremely jealous of the student or group who may be associated with a spiritual teacher. It is amusing to a Hindu, and we think it would be amusing to all Orientals; however, this abnormal idea of a teacher is far from the truth. This is not the principle to be discussed. Yet, when a person tries to study philosophy with the abnormal idea that one teacher can have only one or a few students, he feels a kind of embarrassment. Because that feeling is present the sense of self-respect creates a conflict in the mind that he should not be jealous of that person nor should he express jealousy because the person is a student of a particular teacher. Our spiritual philosophy or mystical training convinces us that we must not express jealousy or envy if we want to be spiritual. This creates a natural conflict in us. Suspicion, and other such secondary emotions, also create extreme forms of mental and nervous disorders and change our behavior.

Suppose we see or hear many nice things about a person whom we envy. We say: "Oh, yes, he is agreeable; however, he doesn't dress well. He is awkward and stands in this way or that way." We happen to know an interesting person, a prominent man, who is extremely jealous of one of his colleagues. At the same time, the man knows that he should not express jealousy, as it is not becoming of him. This very conflict colors his behavior and causes him to use slandering expressions in order to lower the other person. We have seen it occur repeatedly and it is most unfortunate. This particular individual suffers from the effect of emotional conflict in his mind, behavior, and body. He has become neurotic and has developed serious functional ailments.

Psychologists who are followers of Freud think that conflicts and frustrations are created only in connection with the sex urge or pleasure urge. Adlerians have the idea that conflicts and frustrations are created because of the urge of self-expression or the power urge. Both are far from the truth. They try to associate the conflict with a specific emotion which is regarded by the particular school as the master urge. It has been found through later interpretation and study that such facts were not true. We happen to know an interesting psychiatrist who allowed himself to be analyzed by Freudians who interpreted his case in terms of sex impulses. Adler also analyzed him and tried to explain that difficulties were created by the malfunctioning of or conflict in self-expression. The gentleman himself was not convinced. We had occasion to study his case carefully, and it is our impression that a kind of dissatisfaction with life itself created these disturbances, as he does not have a sound philosophy of life. The elements of self-preservation, knowledge, and companionship are operating in the human mind, and conflicts and frustrations can be created by any one of these primitive instincts.

An individual was persuaded by his parents to take up engineering. He had considerable success; yet he was not happy about it in spite of his position, and he began to have functional ailments. It was found that the type of profession imposed upon him was not satisfactory to his inner nature. He succeeded to the best of his ability, but it did not give him satisfaction. The same situation was found to be true in the case of the psychiatrist previously mentioned; his profession did not satisfy his inner nature, so the symptoms of functional ailments and mental disturbances became operative. It will not be out of place to say that he had a successful profession, well-established social position, normal marriage, and normal children.

Similarly, we find that a person can have conflict created by the knowledge urge. All of these emotions can create a conflict and produce functional ailments. These primitive urges and secondary emotions, prospective as well as retrospective, can have serious effects on our bodies. It has been discovered that the secondary emotions of worry and remorse result in nerve disorders. Headache, heart trouble, and all sorts of pains and aches are created by these emotions. Little do we understand how such inner emotions can cause physical disturbances. Dr. Joseph H. Pratt of the Boston Dispensary says:

Dr. Golden working in the medical clinic of the Boston Dispensary has studied the effect of suggestion in about 300 cases of pain. Often the pain had been continuous and severe for weeks or months. His procedure consists of thrusting a hypodermic needle attached to an empty syringe into the skin of the painful area after it has been painted with iodine for the purpose of sterilizing the skin. Dr. Golden does not tell the patient he is going to remove the pain. As he is preparing for the needle test in the presence of the patient he remarks in a low voice to his assistant, but plainly audible to the patient, how surprising it is that the procedure he is about to employ has removed all pain within a minute or two in 90 per cent of the cases in which he has used it. After the needle has been withdrawn he stands by the patient's side, watch in hand. At the end of thirty seconds he asks how the pain is now and writes down the answer. At the end of a minute the query is repeated. Usually the patient says it is less at the end of thirty seconds and entirely gone after two minutes. In about half the cases the pain returned within twenty-four hours following this treatment by suggestion but sometimes complete relief persisted for weeks and rarely for months.

Dr. Golden's work indicates that apparently pain of psychic origin is common, and furthermore it has demonstrated that this pain is often localized and may occur in persons who present no obvious signs of hysteria or nervousness. . . . The conclusion seems justifiable that a pain removed immediately by mental treatment is probably mental rather than physical in origin but we have found occasionally that organic pain has been abolished by Golden's procedure—in one instance the pain in acute pleurisy and in another epigastric pain in a patient who had a peptic ulcer which later perforated.[2]

A prominent scientist reported to me an interesting case showing how fear can paralyze a person. A businessman went on a pleasure trip with a companion. When they were coming back they were overtaken by a bad snowstorm. The man

[2] Joseph H. Pratt, *The Influence of Emotions in the Causation and Cure of Psychoneuroses* (Philadelphia: J. B. Lippincott Co., 1934), pp. 9-10. Reprinted from *International Clinics*, Vol. IV, Series 44.

almost lost hope of returning home safely. There was strong fear of losing prestige and getting into trouble. When he arrived home, he was paralyzed and could not get out of the car. This man could not be cured medically; even psychiatric treatment could not help him, but he was later cured by prayer and other spiritual methods. The scientist who told this is of the opinion that the man recovered when fear and apprehension of various types, including consciousness of guilt and sin, were removed from his mind. The effect vanished and paralysis disappeared.

Another person has been suffering from ear trouble and has been treated by several ear specialists. The latest diagnosis of a great specialist is that emotional disturbances, dissatisfaction, and unhappiness are affecting the glands and the circulatory system, resulting in this type of ear trouble. According to the specialist, the patient can be cured only when he will have emotional satisfaction. It is observed that he feels well when he is peaceful and not upset.

Dr. Pratt reports that even toothache and other such troubles originate in the emotional life of an individual. This does not mean that toothache is imaginary; but apprehension, worry, disgust, jealousy, and anger disturb the proper functioning of the nerves, and ailments follow. Dr. Alexander makes interesting observations and statements regarding psychosomatic disorders.[3] Today, the majority of prominent physicians are thoroughly convinced that most of our physical ailments are originally functional disorders. Dr. Elihu S. Wing, President of the Rhode Island Medical Society, often detects psychogenic functional disorders, pains, and aches; and he treats the cases accordingly. He definitely suggests that a sound philosophy of life and consequent mental stability are of immense help to the functional cases. Moreover, he and other physicians find that even glandular

[3] Alexander, *The Medical Value of Psychoanalysis*, pp. 188-98.

trouble, like overactivity of the thyroid and other glands, is created and accentuated by emotional causes. We know that many other physicians follow this method and help the patients by establishing mental adjustment and stability. In fact, we happen to be acquainted with the diagnoses made by some of the prominent physicians who definitely suggest this method in cases with functional ailments.

When the mind is troubled, when it has conflicting tendencies and is inharmonious and restless, the whole nervous system will be upset and will not function properly. Glands will be affected, and the circulatory system also will be disturbed. As a result, many ailments arise such as dyspepsia, headache, indigestion, and other difficulties which can easily become chronic. Perhaps many persons would be surprised to learn that some surgical cases were found to be really functional in origin and could have been treated and cured had they been detected in time.

Several years ago we had the interesting experience of interviewing a great surgeon in Boston with regard to a patient who appeared to be a surgical case. Some doctors had diagnosed the condition, which was acute, as duodenal ulcer. The Boston surgeon, after examining the patient and studying X-ray pictures which he had taken, came to the conclusion that the case was really functional, which has since proved to be true. We were told that a certain surgeon had definitely wanted to operate, but the Boston doctor had a different opinion. "Swami," he said to me, "I can operate on this man but it would be cruelty to do so. After the operation I can tell you that he will be all right for a few days. As long as he is in the hospital, as long as he is an invalid, and as long as he does not resume his normal activities he will get on well enough; but the moment he takes up his customary duties, his old ailments will reappear. In other words, as long as he remains quiet, his mind will be at ease and he will be all right; but as soon as he attempts to do his usual work, his mind will be disturbed, and the old symptoms will return. So, Swami, tell him to learn to live." Would you not accept that advice from an eminent surgeon concerning a patient who was supposed to be a surgical case? His words, "tell him to learn to live," have deep significance.

We had a similar experience with another Boston surgeon who was a well-known specialist in cancer and malignant diseases, perhaps the most outstanding scientist in this field in the East. Again the case was supposed to be surgical, but he told me definitely that it was merely functional and not a case of cancer. In other words, it was also a case of nerve disorder. This doctor advised the patient to strengthen his mind. He said that when the nervous system was controlled and strengthened the symptoms of disease would disappear. From these two instances, and other such cases, it is safe to conclude that the claims made by reliable psychotherapeutists and psychiatrists are really valid.

Every emotion has its reaction in the nervous system. For instance, love, sympathy, affection, or high spiritual emotions have a pleasing reaction. Have we not observed that when a mother is extremely irritated and comes into the presence of a sweet, smiling child her whole facial expression changes? We have also seen that when we have been in the presence of a gigantic spiritual personality the whole body was refreshed. We have, on certain occasions, seen people coming to a great spiritual personality with much sorrow and heartache, and after remaining in that presence even for a few minutes the people were changed. There was little talk. Perhaps the holy man said: "Hello, come in" or "How are you?" Perhaps he gave a gentle touch of blessing. It is almost impossible to believe that such things happen, but his smiling and happy presence removed the whole heartache, and the nerves became quiet.

It is also true that when we eat we should have a happy atmosphere and not become excited. We should talk of pleasant things because it helps digestion. Then the nerves function properly and the body remains quiet. On the other hand, when we have violent emotions we find the body shaking. With an outburst of anger the body trembles all over, poison is generated, and we cannot have proper digestion.

We have repeatedly seen that many lives are ruined by conflicts of emotion. Apart from the conflict, the emotions also create functional ailments and mental disturbances if there is a lack of balance. It is interesting to know that the human mind possesses certain powers of establishing a kind of harmony among the primitive emotions. The normal man is one whose emotions are well balanced. As there is always a danger of neurosis, however, we should be constantly alert that we do not lose the balance of the mind. When there is conflict or an extremely strong emotional urge, we often try to repress it either because of our feeling of self-respect or for other reasons.

Many of the Freudians, and even Lord Russell, would have us believe that repression is generally created by the so-called ethical and religious teachings. Some seem to think that religious teachings are responsible for repressions; others are of the opinion that the mind tries to repress painful emotions or experiences; while another group comes to the conclusion that it is not merely the sense of pain that causes repression but the sense of propriety, self-respect, and other such ideas. However, we can safely conclude that it is our very nature to repress disagreeable or unbecoming emotions or urges; and if we observe that our feelings are getting out of hand, we try to repress them. These repressions may be of voluntary or involuntary types.

A psychiatrist told us about the interesting case of his son, who was an officer during the First World War. Whenever he was asked to lead a particular operation, he felt almost paralyzed. He was so nervous about it that his voice was affected and he could not move. Fear of fear was most paralyzing to him; he was afraid lest others notice that he was in that condition. After a few moments, somehow or other he would regain his strength. This happened every time he had to do a particular thing. In this case the fear was so possessive that he wanted to repress it, yet the paralyzing effect was there.

It is true that repression of emotion is harmful and it creates functional ailments. Again, many persons adopt a defense reaction. They want to hide their emotions and they show other attitudes instead. Sometimes people take up what they call substitution. They have a strong emotion of sex or self-expression for which they try to substitute something creative in the form of art, painting, and other such activities. Then they sublimate that particular emotion through music or the arts. It is found that these methods are not permanently successful. When proper conditions or environments are offered, the original urges again become operative. All limitations, all embankments or defenses, so to speak, are washed away. We often observe that when there is a mighty current in the river the little embankments are swept away, creating havoc. Similarly, these emotional urges sometimes become so strong that, if the right stimuli are offered and the environment is favorable, all methods of substitution and sublimation become negligible.

Hindu psychologists, in fact spiritual leaders all over the world, advocate the use of self-control. This does not mean repression, as many psychiatrists and rationalists seem to apprehend. Self-control is based on the understanding and use of higher values of life. Stoics would advise one to control certain tendencies and conditions, knowing they are undesirable yet sometimes feeling helpless in coping with them.

The real spirit of self-control, however, as we advocate it, is based on the changing values of life. When a man learns to eat a better type of food, he has no further interest in an inferior quality. Similarly, when one's mind is in the habit of enjoying higher values, like spiritual understanding and realization, it does not find an interest in the lower tendencies or human urges and instincts.

Some of the Western psychologists, such as McDougall and others, seem to think that the instincts cannot be changed. It is true that instinctive drives are inherent in animals; but they do not seem to realize that man, in spite of his animal nature, is more highly evolved. Man does not live on the instinctive plane. His intellectual achievements prove that he can overcome some of the instinctive drives by cultivation of higher intellectual attitudes. We also observe that man has a still higher nature, a spiritual nature, which includes moral values. When man evolves on the spiritual plane, he completely changes his primitive instincts and urges. Sri Ramakrishna, the great spiritual leader of modern India, gives an appropriate illustration in this connection: "When the new leaves sprout in a palm tree, the old leaves drop off without doing any damage whatsoever to the plant itself." Similarly, when the spiritual nature of man is evolved in the form of love, unselfish service, sacrifice, and other such noble tendencies, his primitive urges drop off. In fact, his instincts are changed completely. It will not be out of place to say that even an animal·changes its instinctive nature when it is domesticated and kept in a spiritual and harmonious atmosphere. We know a case in which a dog and a deer actually lived together in a spiritual place with towering spiritual personalities and did not express their natural enmity. They completely overcame their primitive instincts and lived as friends. We also know that a cat and a mouse lived in the same place without showing any instinctive enmity toward each other. Many domestic animals change their primitive urges when they are retrained and kept in a harmonious atmosphere. Even ferocious animals change their natures under the influence of great spiritual personalities, as we know in the life of St. Francis of Assisi and also some great Hindu teachers.

"To die to live" is to overcome the lower self and lower directions of the emotions in order to manifest the higher nature and higher values of life. Then one expands and becomes absorbed in higher phases of experience. Consequently, the lower tendencies die out. The spirit of self-control can be clearly understood from the evolution of human nature. A child is, no doubt, absorbed in dolls, but when maturity comes he enjoys higher emotional expressions far more than the satisfactions he found in the dolls. When a person grows up, he seeks the highest values of spiritual culture in love, unselfishness, and other such elevated ideals. His nature goes through a transformation. When a man constantly thinks and acts on the higher planes of existence and manifests higher values in his activities, and when he is in a state of divine realization, his whole system is thoroughly changed and transformed. Selfish attitudes and gratifications are naturally to be controlled in order that we may expand and gradually become universal. Human beings possess a peculiar relationship with God and until they have a definite realization of that connection there is no peace. There is an inherent tendency in man to be universal. "Joy is in the Infinite, not in the finite," the *Upanishads* (Hindu scriptures) tell us. This explains why a man cannot help seeking religious unfoldment. Knowing these basic principles of human nature, we cannot conclude that self-control is to be construed as repression.

The most outstanding urge in people is the search after the abiding spirit or God. There is an inherent desire in every man to experience the abiding spirit, and until he reaches that goal there is no hope for real peace of mind. This may seem to be a strong declaration, but when we think of God we find that the primitive instincts are reduced to the master urge for bliss. We may have a strong feeling for self-expression or any other urge, yet, when we carry it out, we are not satisfied. The successful physician and psychiatrist, who was previously mentioned, has a fine family and home, yet he remains dissatisfied. Something is missing; something is lacking. You and I know and have found that when people have led a life of success they very frequently have no real satisfaction inside themselves in spite of their so-called expression and position.

Until the innate urge for bliss is fulfilled and understood, there is no satisfaction in life. Frustrations cannot otherwise be successfully eliminated. We do not realize that we possess in the soul a mine of bliss. We go here and there seeking self-expression and self-preservation, while the whole thing is within us. Sri Ramakrishna illustrates this with an interesting example. The musk deer develops musk around its navel. When it matures, the deer gets its fragrance and searches everywhere for it; the foolish deer does not know that he possesses this fragrance all the time. We, too, do not realize that the mine of joy is within us, and we seek happiness in outside activities and pursuits. When we find inner joy, the other emotions are established in their proper places. It does not mean that you or I have to go to a monastery or convent to understand the guiding spirit. In this world we must make Him the center of life, and then we will find the emotions will be well balanced. The individual members of a symphony orchestra have direction and guidance from the conductor. If the influence of the conductor is withdrawn and the different players are allowed to lose co-ordination and co-operation, there will be conflict, confusion, and chaos. Similarly, if the guiding principle of divine power or spiritual value of life is withdrawn, there will be inevitable chaos in the life of a man resulting in conflict and frustration. But as long as we have God as the center of our lives we will find that the emotions of primitive and secondary types will be harmonized and integrated, and all conflicts will be dissolved. Life will be a wonderful expression of joy and happiness. This conclusion can be verified by the study of the lives of men and women who have attained a high level of spiritual realization.

CHAPTER IV

The Subconscious Mind

UNTIL about fifty years ago, almost all psychologists and philosophers in the West were interested only in the understanding of the conscious state of mind, while the study of the subconscious, or unconscious, was practically neg-lected. Although there have been a few references to the sub-conscious in the writings of psychologists, they do not give us complete understanding of it. In the West the study of the subconscious mind was started by Charcot and his student Janêt, the great French psychologists. They made a study of some mental cases and, in the course of their observation, they realized that the conscious states of mind and behavior of man depend greatly on something that is not known to the individual or to others. During their experiments in hypnotism[1] they gathered materials which convinced them that the mind has not only a conscious state but also a hidden state, the subconscious, which is the determining factor of man's conscious activities. Janêt's successor, Freud, made a great discovery of the inner states of the mind which are not known to the average man and yet are powerful and ex-tremely dynamic in changing his conscious activities and behavior.

The study of the subconscious is not one of mere scholastic

[1] Mesmer started the practice of hypnotism (then known as mesmerism). Dr. Braid, an English surgeon, later began to use it under the name of hypnotism.

interest or philosophical implication; it is vitally connected
with the personality of man. We cannot determine the behavior of an individual unless we have a thorough understanding of his subconscious states of mind. The larger portion of the mind is not known to anyone. It remains submerged, like the iceberg, under the conscious realm. Nevertheless, the subconscious mind is more powerful and dynamic
than the conscious mind. According to many of the Western
psychologists, the subconscious mind determines human
behavior; in fact, the conscious activities of an individual
are wholly determined by the subconscious states. Often
when we act in a particular way we ask ourselves: "Why do
I behave like this?" The reason why we cannot answer this is
that the behavior is not caused by our conscious mind but by
the power of the subconscious. Many Western psychologists
conclude that this subconscious really makes up the conscious,
which is nothing but a few bubbles that arise on the surface
of the mind. Hindus explain the subconscious by saying that
it is the repository of the *samskaras* or past impressions
which make up the main contents of the subconscious mind.
In his exposition of *Karma Yoga*, Swami Vivekananda says:

> Every work that we do, every movement of the body, every
> thought that we think, leaves such an impression on the mind-
> stuff, and even when such impressions are not obvious on the
> surface they are sufficiently strong to work beneath the surface,
> subconsciously . . . each man's character is determined by the
> sum total of these impressions.[2]

Thus we see that the study of the subconscious is of vital importance. We cannot have an understanding of a person and
his behavior until we understand his inner states of mind.

When we study the mind we see that it is the arena of conflicting emotions and feelings, ideas and sentiments. It is the

[2] *Works*, I, 52.

battlefield of our mental states and processes. It contains the conscious thoughts and feelings within the scope of our awareness as well as the subconscious ideas and emotions of which we are oblivious. Often thoughts and tendencies arise from the subconscious realm which the conscious mind tries to submerge or repress. This tendency to repress is called "defense reaction." Frequently we may have impulses, emotions, or feelings that we know are unworthy, unwise, or unpleasant, and we endeavor to suppress them, to keep them under control, thinking that by doing this we have driven them away. Unfortunately, they have not gone. They remain in the realm of the subconscious and are preserved within our inner mental life. When an opportunity occurs, they will rise to the surface and become active. If they are very strong, and yet are kept in a repressed state for a long time, they may create nerve disorders, neurotic conditions, or an unbalanced state of mind. Repressed emotions and feelings, unconscious urges and desires create functional diseases. They are at the root of many ailments and maladies. Again, the repressing process may occur on the subconscious plane. Sometimes subconscious feelings, ideas, and complexes do not allow freedom of expression or the functioning of urges on the conscious plane. Such restriction is called "censorship" by modern psychoanalysts.

There is another method of dealing with forbidden or unfulfilled desires and repressed tendencies which the psychoanalysts call "sublimation." This takes place when the mind makes a conscious effort to substitute one emotion for another or to give an urge another mode of expression. The emotion, while still being utilized, is diverted from the course that it would naturally have taken; and the vital energy, or libido, is directed into other channels. In this way the object of desire is replaced gradually by another ideal, and its motivating power is absorbed in the attainment of another purpose. Suppose a man has a very strong urge or instinct that pulls him toward a certain course of action, but he tries to direct it to some other channel. Perhaps he will turn it to artistic or literary creation or to some other constructive pursuits, believing that by so doing he will be able to remove his original strong impulse. Many persons think that this process will enable them to control submerged or subconscious emotions and sentiments. They try to direct their forbidden impulses to some higher form of expression. In some cases sublimation becomes creative and constructive; sometimes it gives new light to a man in mental conflict.

There are people, however, who do not take up the process of sublimation but resort to liquor, narcotics, or other habits in order to forget frustrated desires, mental conflicts, and disturbances. No doubt they are trying to escape from agonizing conditions, but this is not the way out. The relief they get is only temporary, for they have merely exchanged a forbidden, repressed, or unsatisfied desire for something more dangerous. Although alcohol and drugs may release the mind temporarily from the pain of its frustrated hopes and longings by giving it false stimulation, forgetfulness, or pleasant physical sensations, the ultimate effects upon the brain and nervous system are deadly. The desire for liquor or narcotics will become more and more imperious, until torture is suffered in trying to satisfy these cravings. Also, the original cause of the addiction to these habits has not been removed. It will remain in the mental background to torment and incite one to further indulgence. A study of the persons who become slaves of drugs or alcohol will convince anyone that the will power is gradually weakened and destroyed and emotional balance and control are lost. The whole nervous system, both voluntary and involuntary, becomes seriously affected with the consequent development of functional ailments. While the process of sublimation can often help individuals in solving their emotional problems, this other method of escape never does. On the contrary, it causes extreme disintegration of the mind.

Modern psychoanalysts claim that neither defense reaction nor sublimation is sufficiently strong to eliminate our inner conflicts. Instead, they may actually cause complexes. It is often true that defense reactions and censorship are responsible for repressions and the creation of complexes. Repressions are very harmful. Hindu psychologists, as well as the psychiatrists of the West, agree that repressed tendencies are at the root of fear complexes and sometimes of superiority, inferiority, and sex complexes, as well as of other neurotic conditions. Sublimation, however, can be effective if employed with right understanding. All complexes are actually created by the tendencies in the subconscious mind that are repressed by conscious thought or feeling, censorship exerted upon the conscious from the subconscious plane, or by certain unconscious tendencies. Herein lies the utility of psychotherapy.

Through psychotherapy, attempts are made to reveal subconscious mental states and processes, thoughts, urges, and desires. The claim is made that most of the mental, nervous, and functional diseases can be cured if a person can only unearth his hidden desires, emotions, and complexes. The moment they are uncovered and recognized by the patient, that very moment the problem of a neurotic condition or unbalanced mental state will be solved. According to many psychoanalysts, the natural expression of repressed urges and emotions will cure the suppressed tendencies, putting an end to the neurotic state. They insist that expression must be given to the primitive instincts or urges of man. In fact, unexpressed love or hatred must be released and directed to the physician. Some are of the opinion that this very release

and expression often relieve the mental tension and establish
a mental balance.

There are various methods by which psychoanalysts try to
restore a patient to a normal state of mind, such as suggestion and analysis. These methods are not mutually exclusive
but are considered separately for convenience. Suggestion
itself has two forms. First, it may be given from the outside
—that is, by the analyst or doctor. If the patient accepts the
suggestion, he endeavors to absorb it into his system, thereby
establishing a harmonious state of mind. The suggestion is
meant to act upon the mind to eliminate conflict between a
strong urge and some other tendency. Of course, this sug-
gestive method must be based upon a "transference" relationship between the doctor and patient. There must be a
transference of feeling; otherwise, the suggestion given will
not be accepted or assimilated, and there will be no effective
result. Transference between the doctor and patient is, therefore, essential to psychotherapy. It is interesting to note what
Dr. Carl Binger says in this connection in his recent book,
The Doctor's Job. The chapter on "The Relationship between Doctor and Patient" is extremely helpful for both
physicians and psychotherapeutists. Dr. Binger definitely
feels that there must be a friendly relationship between doctor and patient. He says: "Its importance lies in the fact that
the physician's effectiveness, his power to heal, depends in
good measure upon the inwardness of this relationship."[3]
He shows that the recovery of patients from various illnesses
is affected by the relationship with the doctor. Then he says:
"I am noting the addition of a new instrument to the doctor's medical bag—the instrument is *trained* human understanding. Without it some of our drugs and tests and gadgets
may prove egregiously useless."[4]

[3] Binger, *The Doctor's Job,* p. 43.
[4] *Ibid.,* p. 51.

Hindu psychologists are of the opinion that there must be a harmonious relationship or friendship between the teacher (*Guru*) and the student or psychologist and client, whichever the case may be. The student or client must be in a receptive mood in order to get durable results from the help given by the psychologist. A mere release of emotional tension may be temporarily helpful and consoling to the distressed mind, or a sympathetic and friendly chat relieves the pain of frustration and mental conflict, yet neither has a permanent value in the integration of mind or in resolving the emotional conflicts and tension. Therefore, the Hindu psychologists insist that not only must the client or student have harmonious feeling toward the psychologist but he should also be in a receptive and submissive mood. On the other hand, the psychologist must be a man of integration in order to be of real help. Furthermore, he must be established in the higher principles of religion.[5] That is to say, he must not only have intellectual or theological understanding of religion but he must also be thoroughly established in the practical application of religious principles in his emotional reactions. Moreover, he must have unification of thought, emotion, and will.

In its second form, suggestion is given by the person himself. A man may realize, either by self-analysis or through some other means, that his mental dissatisfaction and conflict are creating nerve disorders, mental agitation, irritation, worries, sleeplessness, and consequent functional disturbances. He may also find that he cannot control his emotions so he tries to give his mind some constructive, harmonizing, and unifying suggestion in the form of an ideal or a philosophy of life. If he can train his mind accordingly, he can himself establish a balanced mental condition and restore his mind to a normal state. By so doing, he can remove neu-

[5] *Works*, III, 50-51.

rotic conditions and nerve ailments. Hindu psychologists strongly advocate this method. It may be said, in this connection, that advanced stages of neurotic cases need external help, encouragement, and inspiration. If employed with right understanding, this autosuggestion can be powerful in determining and harmonizing a man's activities.

By the other method, analysis, the doctor tries to study the patient's mind, allowing him to talk freely and give what is called "free association," listening carefully to the story, making observations, and noting all details. In the early days, Janêt hypnotized the person to bring out the hidden tendencies of the mind. Freud also made use of hypnotism, but not finding it efficacious he gave it up. Hindu teachers consider hypnotism in any form to be positively harmful. The superimposition of the will of another, no matter how well-intentioned, weakens the will power of the patient. A man under hypnotic influence loses initiative and the power of decision, and the effect is disastrous to mental harmony and balance. One absolutely needs to develop his own will power if he would be free from mental disturbances.

Freud's method was to allow the patient to tell his own life story, and it is this method which is followed generally by many psychoanalysts today. Many Freudians are of the opinion that the mind establishes stability in the process of analysis when the patient discovers himself and his inner life and tendencies. Others say that the analyst must make a decision for the patient. When the individual is encouraged to talk and the hidden complex is discovered, the analyst often prescribes some helpful suggestion, thought, or constructive idea. In the study and analysis of cases, analysts often find that a man cannot fully remember the details of his life and so they give a little help. In general, it is safe to say that when the analysis is finished, according to Western psychotherapy, the physician or analyst really knows how the patient's mind is reacting. Many cases have been helped by this method, which is used especially for emotional disorders. It is said that many persons gain a balance of the repressed urges, and conflicts in the mind are also dissolved automatically by this method.

Cases of emotional disorder due to conflicts and frustrations are perhaps the most usual types that a psychiatrist is called upon to treat. Many persons misuse or misdirect their emotions for various reasons—existing circumstances, misjudgment, error, family compulsion, social tradition, and many other such causes. They become dissatisfied with their lives because of changes, loss of friends, fluctuations in their own financial conditions, death of a dear one, and even because of the inevitable changes in their own physical health, such as when youth and vigor are followed by infirmity and old age. This dissatisfaction causes their minds to become unsettled, and it is only when the disrupting tendencies can be brought into balance that the conflict can be removed. Then functional and nerve diseases caused by the neurotic condition can be successfully treated.

Analysis can often be useful in determining what should be one's vocation in life. Perhaps a man has an idea that he is fitted for some special work, engineering, for example, yet after taking it up he becomes dissatisfied. This unrest may create a peculiar mental condition which in turn develops into a psychosis. He becomes morose and taciturn and may even begin to show abnormal tendencies. Through analysis the psychiatrist can find out the true nature of the man's mind and the real talents, the natural gifts or tendencies, that are being repressed. In the light of this understanding, he can suggest the vocation which will give the needed expression to the patient's abilities and bring him satisfaction. When he is doing the job for which he was really fitted, and which his subconscious mind really wanted, the neurotic condition is automatically removed and a healthy mental state established.

Professor Carl R. Rogers contributes interesting and useful ideas in the realm of psychotherapy in his book *Counseling and Psychotherapy*. He and many others in America advocate insight by the client as the most effective part of psychotherapy. His use of the word "counseling" is also well chosen and effective. According to him and others, the client should be helped by the counselor to have insight into the cause of the mental disturbance. Professor Rogers thinks that the client should develop such insight during the course of counseling and adopt a method of orientation to life. He says:

> The client's insight tends to develop gradually and proceeds in general from less to more significant understanding. It involves the new perception of relationship previously unrecognized, a willingness to accept all aspects of the self and a choice of goals. Following these new perceptions of self and this new choice of goals come self-initiated actions which move toward achieving the new goals. . . . They create new confidence and independence in the client.[6]

Professor Rogers comes to the conclusion that the directive suggestions in the course of analysis or counseling are not so successful. They are often incompletely done or rejected.

There have been cases of autognosis in which a person by self-analysis discovered his own hidden complexes and urges by examining the incidents of his life. In a sense, it is a reliving of the life itself. Instead of going to a psychiatrist, some persons (though only a few) succeed in recognizing their subconscious tendencies through introspection, and then they themselves try to establish balance in them. Most of the modern analytical psychiatrists do not give much

[6] Carl R. Rogers, *Counseling and Psychotherapy* (Boston: Houghton Mifflin Co., 1942), p. 216.

recognition to this method. However, it is mentioned by Dr. William Brown in his book, *Science and Personality*.

Dr. Karen Horney's book on Self-analysis should be specially mentioned. She emphasizes the use of self-analysis as an effective method of psychotherapy. Her arguments in favor of it are refreshing and convincing. She says:

> But even apart from such blatant reasons, certain gains are beckoning to those who are capable of self-analysis which are more spiritual in character, less tangible, but not less real. These gains can be summarized as an increase of inner strength and therefore of self confidence.[7]

Some psychiatrists believe that neither autognosis nor heterognosis is sufficient for establishing harmony among conflicting urges and thereby restoring the normal condition of mind and nerves—especially Adler, Jung, and some others who realize that mere knowledge of the subconscious urges and the causes of repression cannot restore mental balance. The patient needs definite educational training according to Adler, and religious training according to Jung, Brown, and others.

The Hindus strongly advocate the method of self-analysis. They specially emphasize the religious methods of discipline in restoring a man to mental wholeness. In this form of self-analysis, no doubt, one discovers his hidden tendencies but he also synthesizes the mind. According to the Hindu view, not only must one analyze one's own self but at the same time one must reconstruct his life. One must build up a sound philosophy and try to mold his life accordingly. The practice of concentration is particularly helpful. We observe that many disintegrated minds are synthesized by the combined methods of self-analysis and concentration. A mere discovery of mental conflict, by either the Freudian method of psycho-

---

[7] Karen Horney, *Self-Analysis* (London: Kegan Paul, 1942), p. 36.

analysis, Rogers' insight, or self-analysis, does not integrate the mind. Our experience proves it is the practice of concentration[8] that brings out hidden mental forces which reconstruct and integrate the whole mind. We can illustrate the effect of the combined methods of insight and practice of concentration and cite many cases in which it was successful. We have also seen persons who were analyzed by Freudians and others. They had insight and understood the causes of their mental disturbances, yet they were not capable of synthesizing their disintegrated minds as they did not have the power of concentration and unified will. Therefore, the Hindus feel that training is an essential part of mental orientation. In fact, this training brings out the latent power in the mind and creates hope and self-confidence, as we shall discuss in later chapters.

Many psychiatrists give great importance to the analysis and interpretation of dreams in the understanding of the subconscious. Freud and his followers lay great emphasis upon this. According to them, dreams are really created by repressed urges, although these may only appear symbolically. By understanding and interpreting the symbols in dreams one can understand the true nature of an underlying urge as well as its intensity. Some psychotherapeutists depend upon this method, but when the different schools of applied psychology try to analyze the symbols in dreams and the basic causes and principles of neurosis they differ widely and find no agreement. Freudians trace everything to the sex impulse or conflict of "life" and "death" urges, while followers of Adler would interpret the same dream in terms of the urge to power. Professor McDougall had his own dreams analyzed by authorities of different schools and found that different causes were attributed to the same dream, according to the theories advanced by the different psychiatrists. He said:

[8] The practice of concentration will be explained in the chapter on " Meditation."

I conclude then that Freud's formula for the interpretation of dreams may be true of some dreams, more especially of some dreams of neurotics . . . but there is no sufficient ground for trying to force the interpretation of every dream to fit the formula.[9]

It is undeniable that many persons find satisfaction and relief when their difficulties are explained to them in the light of the sex urge or the urge of self-expression, but it would be unpardonable to say that either impulse is the key to the whole truth of the nature of man or that every dream can be interpreted by it alone. What is true with regard to the understanding of dreams is also applicable to the other methods of psychoanalysis in general, whatever may be the name of the particular school and its methods.

Hindu psychologists do not accept the theory that all dreams are created by causal relationship with past experiences or that they are determined by repressed urges of sex or self-expression; nor do they try to explain all dreams in the light of mental repressions, wish fulfillment, and other such causes. Dreams need not necessarily be created by inhibitions, repressed conscious or subconscious urges, or even by impressions from past thoughts and actions, although it is true that many dreams do come from these causes. Dreams are not always retrospective. To illustrate this we can relate dream experiences of some of our intimate friends in the West. For the sake of authenticity we will relate a few of the most reliable dreams, which were verified. We are deliberately relating the cases from American sources.

A friend of ours had a most amazing dream just before the Vedanta Society of Boston acquired its present building. We had been negotiating through a real estate company to buy this property, and one morning we requested our friend,

[9] William McDougall. *Outline of Abnormal Psychology* (London: Methuen, 1926), p. 186.

who was interested in the negotiations, to make an offer for the house. She said: "Swami, if I am to make an offer I shall give the amount of which I dreamt." It was almost less than half of the sale price. We felt that the Society would lose this opportunity to have the place if such an offer were made. However, our friend insisted on it, and when we went to Boston the offer was given to the real estate agent. He was vexed and almost decided to drop the matter without relaying the offer to the owner. We finally persuaded him to take a check with the offer to the owner, who would have the choice of refusing it. The next morning the real estate agent telephoned and told our friend that her dream was true, as the owner had accepted the offer. The house was acquired as indicated previously in the dream.

Another friend had an unusual dream of a certain section of Boston being burned. It was so vivid that she could describe even the position of the flagpoles and other details of the locality, which she had never seen in her life. The next morning the newspaper reported a huge conflagration in Boston, and upon inquiry it was found that all details of the dream were true.

A friend of ours dreamed of the critical illness of a Swami just before it occurred. The details of that sickness as well as the process of recovery shown in the dream were wholly verified by the developments and later events of the case. We can relate a number of such progressive dreams about the future which were thoroughly verified by later events, so it is a mistake to think that dreams are all causally related and retrospective.

Some dreams are progressive and creative; others, again, give evidences of spiritual unfoldment. Still other leave tremendous impressions upon the mind amounting to spiritual joy and realization. Jung is of the opinion that some dreams are progressive. He relates many instances in which they gave knowledge of future events.[10] Hindus also believe in the prophetic nature of some dreams—that they may sometimes give indications or foreshadowings of the future, as in the cases mentioned above.

Dreams can also be in the form of religious instructions. We know authentic instances in which men and women received definite spiritual instructions in a dream. Some have even received initiation (symbolical names of God and other spiritual practices) from their spiritual teachers in dreams. The *mantras* (names of God) which they received were never known previously to them. These words constituted completely new knowledge. Other instructions received in dreams in the form of spiritual practices, methods of work, and ways of life were unique and uplifting. The contents of such dreams cannot be traced to any previously experienced events or to any form of personal or "racial" unconscious, as Professor Jung would want us to believe. The dreamers have had unique experiences which cannot be traced to the race in which they were born. Some did not even know the language or meaning of the *mantra* (name of God) until this was later given to them by the teacher. The spiritual instructions which students or devotees get in dreams indicate not only their spiritual inspiration but also their prophetic nature. On the basis of these known experiences we again say that there are many dreams which do not originate in the unconscious or in physical disorders.

Apart from the future understanding of ordinary events, there are dreams, as we explained previously, which are definitely a part of spiritual realization. Their effect remains permanent and changes the course of life. Again, some dreams solve many metaphysical and spiritual problems of

[10] Carl G. Jung, *Modern Man in Search of a Soul* (London: Kegan Paul, 1935), chap. I.

life, giving definite and illuminating knowledge and high emotional satisfaction.

According to modern psychiatrists, man has certain primitive or primary instincts which must be allowed expression if he is to be normal and well balanced. However, psychiatrists do not agree on the relative importance of these urges or which is the most fundamental or predominant. Freud and his followers interpret the activities of man in terms of the sex urge, although of late they take a broader point of view. They try to show that the sex instinct is the motivating power behind all expression from the simplest forms, as in the seeking of pleasure, to the greatest achievements in the arts or other creative activities. Religious experiences to them are but the sex tendency translated into spiritual emotions. Some even go so far as to say that the idea of God Himself has its origin in sex. They analyze a man's whole nature and mental outlook from this point of view, feeling that if anything is wrong it can be traced directly to this fundamental impulse. The repression of the sex urge is to them unhealthy and dangerous. They declare that it is at the root of complexes, neuroses, and other unhappy and unbalanced mental conditions, and even of religious enthusiasm. As we mentioned in the first chapter, Freud later changed his theory concerning the primary urge. He came to the conclusion that man's activities can be traced to both the "life" and the "death" instincts, or sex and suicide urges, and that man's behavior is motivated by the interaction of these urges. Orthodox Freudians, like Karl A. Menninger, give an unhappy (almost repugnant) interpretation of life.[11] While we do not agree with this generalization, we do give credit for many notable achievements in analyzing mental cases that are suited or responsive to interpretation by the sex impulse.

[11] Karl A. Menninger, *Love Against Hatred* (London: Harrap, 1942), and *Man Against Himself.*

Yet we make bold to say that they have made unfortunate and uncalled-for generalizations from some abnormal cases.

It is interesting to note that Adler takes a different view from Freud regarding the fundamental urge in man. It is his belief that the dominant instinct in man is the urge to power, or self-expression, and he does not agree that it is the sex urge which lies at the root of man's activities. He teaches that man has a strong tendency to express himself, to exert power, and to crave for the fulfillment of all his possibilities. When this is denied, thwarted, or repressed, difficulties are bound to arise. When a man cannot express himself, when he cannot exert power, or, as in some cases, when he cannot dominate others, he feels limited, imprisoned, and crushed. Adler claims that this is the real root of mental unbalance.

It is true that men have a desire for power, often for ruling over others, and it cannot be denied that there is a strong tendency toward self-expression in everyone. When this urge is unusually strong and intense, or when there is not sufficient outlet, the mind does become dissatisfied and consequently upset; and nerve troubles, complexes, or other disturbances arise. Yet as we study the whole nature of man, as we analyze the whole mind scientifically, we do not think that either the Freudian school or the Adlerian school is really correct. Each makes a valuable contribution, no doubt, and each is helpful in certain cases, but they do not go far enough. They arbitrarily generalize from the study of a few pathological cases, as previously explained. By observation and careful study we discover that there are other primary instincts to be reckoned with in the nature of man besides the sex impulse or the will to power. For instance, there is the instinct of self-preservation, accompanied by the powerful emotion of fear. Many human activities are motivated by this urge. How quickly fear will arise the moment a man thinks his safety is threatened or when he suspects that something is about to destroy him! Many will cling to life on almost any terms, and it is common knowledge that a sudden panic can transform a cultured, well-behaved group into a mass of struggling brutes. It is not the sex urge or the will to power that is always at the root of mental disorders. The instinct of self-preservation, too, under certain conditions, can create difficulties.

In this connection we happened to study a certain case carefully. It had nothing to do with sex or power urges. A woman developed a psychogenic neurosis. She was treated by different analysts but could not be cured, although at times she was helped a little. When she was a child, certain teachings created an abnormal fear of punishment as a result of certain wrongdoings. This was impressed so much on the child's mind that when she grew up she could not shake it off. For a long time she lived a fairly successful life in business and marriage, but owing to changes in the circumstances of her life her security was threatened. This brought out the old fear and apprehension which had been forgotten until she was about thirty years of age. A serious mental and nerve disorder was created, and the woman had difficulty even in crossing the street without a companion. She was restored to a normal state by a proper understanding of the higher values of life and higher nature of man. With this understanding she found a meaning in life and its utility. We happen to know that psychoanalysis and general autognosis or insight did not cure her. Autognosis with the help of creative and constructive suggestion, as opposed to the destructive and negative childhood suggestion, was immensely helpful. We had to give her a sound philosophy of life and emphasize the higher nature of man. Mental training and exercises gradually began to synthesize her mind. Steady practice of concentration brought out latent inner strength and created self-confidence and conviction; the mind was reconstructed and normality established.

We know many persons who are afflicted by maladjustment in the urge of self-preservation and other urges and emotions. We can cite many cases to prove that all the emotions under certain conditions can become sources of trouble. After World War I some eminent scientists, Dr. William Brown and others, observed cases that had become neurotic —not because of repression of the sex impulse or need for self-expression, but because of fear complexes. Some patients were known to have developed psychoses, even insanity, through fear of war and destruction. Many that were thought to be cases of shell shock had not actually experienced the shock but had developed the symptoms from fear of it.

Again, the gregarious instinct in man is strong. Man seeks companions; he wants to have friends around him. He feels loneliness when there is no one near. This desire for social relationships is one of the primary urges, as we explained in the chapter on "Emotion." It is not to be identified with the sex instinct, as Freud tried to claim by having recourse to unwarrantable imagination, nor is it due to the wish for power or the desire to domineer over others, as Adler would have us believe. Man wants friends primarily because he has joy in their company. He does not seek them merely for protection and the expression of sex or power, but rather for the exchange of thoughts and emotions to share his ideas and experiences. The repression or denial of this communal impulse can often derange a man's mind. It has been found by observation that many persons will become mentally unbalanced if left alone for a long period of time. When people cannot have friends or companions, when they must live in isolated places such as on a desert, marooned on an island, or in solitary confinement, they tend to become queer and eccentric, if not positively insane. There are various reasons for this, but the fundamental cause is the repression of the normal instinct for companionship. There are, of course, some exceptional persons who do not care for social life owing to an inner fear, the result of early training by their parents, or because of other conditions and circumstances; but these are rare cases. There are also persons who live an intense inner life, not because they have the selfish nature of an introvert but because of a profound interest in the realization of higher things—spirituality or truth or God. Men engaged in scientific research, great spiritual leaders, scholars, and others of a like nature will prefer to remain alone for long periods of time. They have deep satisfaction in their pursuits and do not depend on social contacts for a happy life.

There is also another instinct in man known as the cognitive instinct. This is the urge to know. Man wants to understand himself and his surroundings; he wants to analyze and discover the truth about the things that he sees. He shows this tendency even as a little child by asking questions and showing interest in the world about him. He is not satisfied with knowing that a thing exists. He wants to find out how and why. This cognitive instinct cannot be interpreted by either the Freudian or the Adlerian theories of primitive urges. If this impulse is unduly accentuated or is not in harmony with other mental tendencies, it also can create disorder. For instance, if a man has only a limited possibility for intellectual unfoldment yet has developed an abnormal desire for it, he will create a neurotic condition, just as in the case of other unbalanced and unsatisfied urges. An abnormal desire for knowledge that is frustrated can create inferiority and superiority complexes and other forms of mental disorder.

After studying the interpretation of the subconscious mind as given by modern Western psychology, it would

appear to a disinterested person as though the subconscious
were considered more or less as a separate mental force to
regulate what the average person understands as the conscious mind. It would also appear that the subconscious is
the repository of the "dark" forces and repressed tendencies
of man which create abnormalities or neuroses. Then, too,
we find Jung speaking of "race subconscious" which influences the subconscious of individuals. From this we can
gather that at least some modern psychologists are conclud-
ing that the subconscious mind contains not only the repressed tendencies of one individual but it is also affected by
the repressed tendencies of those about him.

Hindu psychologists give great stress to inherent tendencies or past impressions (*samskaras*), of which the subconscious consists. These impressions from past thoughts and
actions may be of good, bad, or indifferent quality. They will
accordingly remain in what is known as the subconscious
state of mind in the form of tendencies. They can be revived
as memories and can become powerful factors, determining
in many cases the functionings of the conscious state. To
quote Swami Vivekananda:

If a man continuously hears bad words, thinks bad thoughts,
does bad actions, his mind will be full of bad impressions; and
they will influence his thought and work without his being conscious of the fact . . . he will be like a machine in the hands of
his impressions, and they will force him to do evil. Similarly . . .
when a man has done so much good work and thought so many
good thoughts that there is an irresistible tendency in him to do
good, in spite of himself and even if he wishes to do evil, his
mind, as the sum total of his tendencies, will not allow him to
do so; the tendencies will turn him back; he is completely under
the influence of the good tendencies.[12]

[12] *Works*, I, 52-53.

The mind of an individual also receives impressions from its environment and from the company of others. Professor Jung gives considerable value to the race unconscious.[13] He comes to the conclusion that man's conscious and unconscious mind is greatly influenced by the race unconscious. Hindu psychologists not only teach that the impressions from other minds may be of a passive nature but also that there may be dynamic influences at work, as well as the active transference of thought. Throughout the ages, Hindu teachers have recognized the fact that there is an active influence exerted by the mind of an individual upon the conscious and subconscious states of others. They also are aware of the power of suggestion. To them, the subconscious mind is not merely the repository of past thoughts and actions but also contains the impressions that are received consciously or unconsciously from others. They believe that past impressions may also remain from a previous life.

According to Hindu teachers, the human mind brings with it experiences from past existences, for they believe in the theory of reincarnation.[14] Hindu philosophers and psychologists are of the opinion that the individual soul goes through various stages of life accumulating experiences and it retains latent possibilities of future evolution and unfoldment, just as the seed contains the possibilities of a future tree. Even when the gross body dies, the impressions (samskaras) of past thoughts and actions are preserved in the subtle body. Hindu thinkers maintain that the soul has not only a gross body but also a subtle and a causal body, each performing different functions. In order to understand these three bodies or sheaths, we can conceive of a person and his different layers of outer and undergarments. Every one of

[13] Carl G. Jung, *Integration of Personality*, trans. Stanley Dell (London: Kegan Paul, 1939).

[14] References to the theory of reincarnation may be found in the following sources. *Works*, I, 239, 318, and 330; *Works*, II, 218-20, 224-25; and Swami Abhedananda, *Reincarnation* (Mylapore, Madras: Sri Ramakrishna Math).

them performs a particular function. The gross body of the individual soul functions on a gross plane. The inner instruments (*antahkarana-manah, buddhi, ahamkar,* and *chitta,* as explained in the second chapter), and such other subtle functionings, are in the subtle body. The causal body consists of the subtle impressions and the basic consciousness of I-ness which individualizes the Self. In reincarnation the individual soul returns to this world in a new gross body with those *samskaras* as the basis of what we call tendencies.[15] The unconscious mind contains these impressions. Many of the individual tendencies and temperaments can be better explained by this viewpoint. Reincarnation is prolonged by the expression of urges which are created by the past residuals of thoughts and actions. The cycle of birth and death ceases to exist only when the whole mind, conscious and unconscious, is totally unified and ultimately freed from inordinate longings and urges by complete illumination.

Within the subconscious mind lies the sum total of the experiences, impressions, and tendencies of an individual; and the quality of its influence upon the conscious state, as well as upon the minds of others, will be determined by the quality of these impressions, according to whether or not they are good, bad, or indifferent.[16] But a man need not be a mere creature of his past. The contents of the subconscious mind created by his own past thoughts and actions, as well as by the influence of others, can be changed or transformed by the creating of new *samskaras,* or impressions.[17] By changing the quality of his mental habits in the present, a man can himself direct and determine what his future mental state shall be. By regulating his thoughts and emotions, a man can make for himself new hope and new possibilities.

[15] *Srimad-Bhagavad-Gita,* trans. Swami Swarupananda (Mayavati, Almora, Himalayas: Advaita Ashrama, 1933), chap. II:22.

[16] *Works,* I, 52.

[17] *Yoga Aphorisms of Patanjali.*

There are many persons in the West who think that Hindu religion and philosophy are fatalistic. This is far from the truth. Hindu philosophers and psychologists firmly believe that a man can change his course of life if he has right understanding and works accordingly, thereby creating a new set of *samskaras*, or impressions, by reorienting his life.

CHAPTER V

Will and Personality

OUR emotions, urges, and instincts are inseparably connected with our volition. We wish to express each one of our emotions. When the mind becomes active in its totality, we call it "will." Without this will we cannot translate our ideas or emotions into action or a dynamic state. Consequently, even though we may have lofty ideas and ideals and exalted emotions, they are not effective in our daily lives. Will is of vital importance to every individual. Sometimes we find that when there is conflict and confusion in the subconscious mind the will is not completed. Because of the conflict, urges arise in one direction and then another with the result that neither a single urge nor a set of urges has maximum satisfaction. Thus will is incomplete and loses its power. Few of us realize that our failures in life are caused by an incomplete will. Generally, the popular expression is: "This man has no will power." However, it is a mistake to think that we do not possess will; rather it has not been integrated or completed. The mind is split, and so we fail. We cannot achieve anything unless we have an integrated or unified will. Therefore, its cultivation is vitally important.

In some cases mental disturbances split the personality wholly. Such cases are to be treated medically first. Some of us must have had occasion to notice individuals who often are timid about crossing the street. A few years ago, a friend of ours introduced a person to us who was extremely afraid to go across the street; she was in such a nervous state that she could not perform her daily activities. It was a deplorable state, and we know from personal contact with other cases, and also from the experiences of some of our medical friends, that there are innumerable similar cases in which an individual cannot manage even ordinary functions. Generally, such patients are helped by psychiatrists who can unearth the conflict; when the conflict is dissolved, the mind is allowed to function properly. The dynamic side of the mind becomes operative, and the individual can then carry on normal activities.

That is not all we want, however; we want more in life than the average person. Average men and women, it is true, can conduct their ordinary affairs, yet they are utterly helpless in the expression of their ideals. They pitifully fail to use higher emotions and spiritual ideals in their lives and actions even though they do not lack theoretical understanding of religious philosophy. Christians have studied the teachings of Christ thoroughly, and the followers of other religions study their respective teachings. We do not believe that there is a child who does not understand the basic principles of the teachings of Christ and other great teachers. They all know that "hatred cannot be conquered by hatred but by love." All the lofty principles are known to the people, yet you find that they cannot make those ideals effective. Why? Because they lack will power. The will is completely disintegrated, and consequently they cannot carry out their aims and ideals.

When you observe a child, you realize that he has different ideals at different times. Sometimes he admires a school teacher, sometimes a Sunday school teacher, or one of his parents. Again he admires the other parent and tries to imi-

tate him. The ideals are shifting constantly, and because they
are not thoroughly operative in the child's life his emotions
are not integrated. When a person enters adolescence, if he
has not been trained to unify his ideals, there is a riot of emotions creating conflicts within him. Today, as a result of this
lack of training, adolescent boys and girls are in a bad state
and are unable to put into effect the things they would like
to do. They also lose their balance of mind, as they are easily
influenced by the different persons whom they meet, and
remain unsteady and fickle. For this reason the will must be
developed if we want to have integrated emotions and strong
ideals in our lives; otherwise we will be slaves, not only of
our own desires and emotions, but also of the emotions and
wills of other people.

There is a great deal of confusion in the minds of many
persons regarding the very nature of will, and the difference
between will and desire, or wish, is not understood. In a wish
there is doubt as to whether or not it will be fulfilled. I wish
to be a wealthy man, but I am not sure that I can become
one. I wish to be a saint, but I am not quite sure that it is
possible for me to become one or, if it is possible, for me to
unify my emotions and translate my ideal into action. There
is this lack of conviction in desire or wish, while the primary
condition of will is conviction. Brown, McDougall, and most
of the psychologists are of the opinion that one must have a
dynamic conviction or faith in one's self in order to develop
the will. Hindu phychologists declare that the basic quality
of will is what they call *shraddha*, often translated as "faith."
As Swami Vivekananda says:

The ideal of faith in ourselves is of the greatest help to us. If
faith in ourselves had been more extensively taught and practiced, I am sure a very large portion of the evils and miseries
that we have, would have vanished. Throughout the history of
mankind, if any motive power has been more potent than an-

other in the lives of all great men and women, it is that of faith
in themselves. . . . But it is not selfish faith, because the Vedanta,
again, is the doctrine of Oneness. It means faith in all, because
you are all.[1]

Shraddha is more than faith. It is a conviction of power
and the desire to translate faith into action. When a man has
a conviction that he can express an ideal or emotion, then
alone his mind becomes dynamic. It becomes active in its
totality. When there is no conviction or faith, there is no
possibility of unifying the will. Some of us must have had
the experience that when we are learning to drive an auto-
mobile or ride a bicycle we are likely to become nervous if
we see something ahead of us. If we remain calm and have
the conviction that of course we can pass the obstacle, then
we go ahead with no hesitancy. On the other hand, if we do
not have the conviction that we can pass the car in front of us,
or go around the rock, we find invariably that the will
weakens and we cannot go through the experience without
agony or nervousness, which often results in an accident or
other difficulties. In order to develop and complete the will,
we must have calmness of mind and conviction. Unless a
man utilizes that conviction or *shraddha*, there is no possibility of achieving anything in life.

> The man of faith,
> Whose heart is devoted,
> Whose senses are mastered:
> He finds Brahman [God]. . . .
>
> The ignorant, the faithless, the doubter
> Goes to his destruction.[2]

Another simple habit is essential for the development of
will. We often start things because of our conflicting ideas

---

[1] *Works*, II, 299.

[2] *Bhagavad-Gita*, trans. Swami Prabhavananda and Christopher Isherwood
(Hollywood: The Marcel Rodd Co., 1944), p. 68.

and ideals, divergent desires and longings. Sometimes, we
want to be musicians or mathematicians; again, when we are
with scientific people, we feel inclined to become scientists;
or perhaps we meet a philosopher and wish to be one, too.
For a few days we attend a music school to study to be a
musician, or a Hindu school to become a psychologist or
yogi; and again, we may go to a philosopher to study philosophy. We do not complete anything; and as a result we dis-
sipate our energy, our mental powers are wasted, and our
will is not stimulated and unified. One ought to complete an
action, whatever it is. Perhaps you have started cooking.
Do not leave the place without finishing this cooking. If you
are baking a cake, finish it. Whether it is a good cake or a
bad cake does not matter; complete it. The mind is peculiar;
once you let it run riot or become jumpy you will find it
hard to control. Another peculiarity of the mind is that it
behaves like a child. You may have observed that a child
will often feel its way and try to find out how far it can go
with the mother. If the child finds that the mother allows a
little more margin, he goes still farther; but the moment discipline is imposed he straightens up. Similarly, the mind
tries to feel its way if it is allowed to do so. Then as soon as
you give it discipline such as: "No, you cannot go; you must
finish this music lesson before you can take up anything
else," you will find that when you form the habit of com-
pleting an act, whether motivated by a particular urge, emotion, instinct, or idea, it will then be easier for the mind to
complete successive actions. As a result, the will becomes
unified.

Hindu psychologists emphasize purity and one-pointedness of mind. In order to develop the highest type of will
power, a man must not allow his inordinate emotions to become dominant. He must cultivate higher principles of
ethics, otherwise the body and mind cannot be pure; more-

over, they must be unified and co-ordinated. For the most
part the mind functions through the nervous system, so that
when the nerves are weak the mind is weak and flighty.
Therefore, the Hindus advocate purity of the body, or nervous system. We often observe that the body is tired or lazy,
energetic or active, balanced or regulated, or to use Hindu
terminology; *tamasic, rajasic,* and *sattvic.* When the body or
the nervous system is full of inertia, the mind also becomes
dull. When the body is active, the mind becomes active. On
the other hand, when the body is in a balanced state, the
mind remains peaceful and happy. Of course, these three
states are generally classified according to the predominance
of one or the other. When we say that purity of the body or
nervous system is advocated, we mean that the body should
be kept in a balanced and controlled state, and the extreme
dull and restless states should be overcome. Unless the nervous system is strengthened, ordinary personalities cannot
expect to have strong minds. However, extraordinary personalities who have reached integration of mind through the
practice of concentration can keep their will strong and the
whole mind unified even if the body is weak. Hindu psychologists are of the opinion that the vitality must be conserved by a regulated and controlled life. They also prescribe
a psychological method to strengthen the will.

There are two ways by which the nervous system can be
helped. One is physical, by which certain foods or forms of
vitamins are taken to strengthen the nervous system. This
strengthening through physical means is temporary; for when
the mind has emotional conflicts or unconscious disturbances,
the nerves become weak and shattered in spite of dietetic
regulations. You and I often observe that when we experience violent emotion the nerves are shaken. A man who is
weak or nervous cannot expect to have a dynamic will, for
the mind cannot function in its totality. Consequently, the

will is split. Therefore, Hindus advise that the emotions first be integrated, purified, and unified, and inner conflicts be dissolved in order to strengthen the nerves. When the nerves become strong through mental purification, the will becomes dynamic.

Our vital force[3] generally functions through two central nerve currents, *ida* and *pingala* according to Hindu terminology, or sensory and motor nerve currents according to modern physiological terms. When these two nerve currents, sensory and motor, are allowed to be dissipated, the will becomes weak. The nerve centers and currents can also be overstimulated and exhausted by extreme mental conflicts, frustrations, apprehensions, anxieties, and other such disturbances. The whole nervous system then becomes shattered, and the functioning of the vital force in the system becomes extremely weakened. According to Hindu psychologists, mental and physical energy can be conserved or dissipated as one allows the vital force to function either effectively or improperly. That is also one of the reasons that some of the Hindu teachers prescribe certain forms of rhythmic breathing. Proper breathing exercises relax the whole body, strengthen the nervous system, and conserve the vital force. After all, the subtlest form of the expression of vital force in human physiology is through the respiratory system. When the respiratory system is regulated, the vital force is conserved. As a result, the nerves become strengthened; and when the nerves are strong, the mind is also strong; the mind can function or remain active in its totality. Consequently, the will is dynamic.

Another important method the Hindus prescribe is the practice of concentration and meditation. We shall not discuss meditation elaborately here as it is treated more fully in the following chapter. However, the practice of concen-

[3] *Prana* or the entity which gives energy and power to the system.

tration makes the mind one-pointed. When we try to concentrate, we focus the mind on one object and do not allow it to waver and go here and there. We discipline the mind and compel it to think of one thing at a time. Of course, in the beginning there is a great deal of difficulty in focusing the mind on one object since we have not formed the habit of thinking of only one thing for several minutes. We may have been thinking constantly of different friends or of our children, but the thoughts are successive and constantly changing; they are not one thought. Even though we may have lovely ideas and emotions, they are still not unified and one-pointed when occurring successively. When we think of a child, we do not focus the mind on one particular aspect but rather on different aspects of that child. When we think of our friends, we consider the details of different experiences with them. We seldom visualize a friend and remain absorbed in one of his particular aspects. Hindus advise us to focus the mind on one thing for some time. The result is wonderful; the whole mind and all the mental forces are converged and integrated. To understand this concentration we can think of the rays of the sun. When the rays are diffused, we do not find intensity of heat or light; but when the rays are converged and focused upon one object, we can even set a fire thereby. Similarly, in concentration we focus the whole mind; all the functions of mind are made one-pointed. As a result, it develops into a unified state and the will is integrated.

In order to integrate the will and make the mind one-pointed, another important factor must be considered. We must have an ideal to follow, a unified ideal. When we have that ideal or higher value of life, if the mental states can operate under it, then the mental forces are integrated and conflicts gradually dissolve. The will becomes active in its totality. Take, for instance, the national heroes. They have

E

one ideal, and under it they organize their entire lives. All their mental forces are utilized in that particular service, resulting in great potentiality for action. A man may also be very destructive when all his forces are directed into one channel.

We observe today, in studying the political history of the world, that there are persons who can put their ideals and urges into effect because their minds are unified. If you have national ideals or family ideals as the organizing factor in your life, there will be invariable conflict with other factors. Mere nationalism as an ideal cannot be constructive and synthesizing for humanity at large even though that ideal can unify a man's emotions and make his will dynamic. That kind of unified will is not conducive to human happiness. A family ideal or national ideal as an integrating force can, no doubt, unify mental states yet it always creates conflict among individuals, families, or nations resulting in feud, conflict, confusion, war, and destruction. The pages of the world's history are full of such discord and disturbance ultimately leading men, who have integrated the will with those ideals, to extreme forms of unhappiness and destruction. Such narrow and limited ideals cannot create a healthy state of mind.

The Hindu psychologists and some of the Western psychologists advise us to take the universal ideal, or ideal of God, as the constructive factor in developing the will. When God is taken as the unifying factor, the integrating element, or the ideal of life, all emotions, thought processes, and mental states are unified; the integrated will then operates only for the good and happiness of all and not for the destruction or conflict of anyone. All the different families and nations can be unified in the universal existence of God with the knowledge that they all are veritable manifestations of the Absolute, or children of God. When a person takes up this universal ideal as the highest value of life, he spontaneously removes the cause of conflict by eliminating divergence of interest among individuals and groups and by unifying all in God. Personal ambitions and interests are subordinated and harmonized for the good and happiness of all. For this reason, the practice of concentrating on an ideal is the best way to bring out the hidden power that we possess. This point will be more elaborately discussed in the later chapters.

Extrasensory perceptions of various types are attained by the unified will; in fact, mystic experiences and superconscious realizations can be had only when the will is integrated. We also know that the unified will has a tremendous influence on the body. Hindu psychology explains how the involuntary actions of the body can be controlled by the developed will. It has been proved by many persons in India that the involuntary actions of muscles can be kept under control, and we know people who have achieved unusual control over the elementary functionings of the human body. There are persons who can also change the rhythm and tempo of the circulatory system with mental control. Human appetites, such as hunger and thirst, can be appeased by the will; in fact, physical ailments can also be removed. We often hear of mental healing. It is true that there are many fraudulent cases, yet there are also many authentic cases of mental healing all over the world. They are often known in the West as miracles. Dr. Alexis Carrel has recorded some of these miraculous cases, and we, too, have witnessed such happenings. We also know that some persons with tremendous will power can control even the laws of nature. This factor will be discussed in the chapter on the effect of "Meditation."

It is well known to the Christian world that St. Francis of Assisi developed stigmata. The real explanation is that St.

Francis wholly unified his mind in Christ in such an in-
tensive way that he even physically identified himself with
Christ. There are many incidents in the life of St. Francis
which are direct results of integrated will. We have heard of
a nun in Bavaria, Germany, who also developed certain
physical characteristics of Christ. We are also told that another nun in Rome shows bodily symptoms every Good
Friday. These can be explained by the understanding of the
higher laws of mind.

When we study the life of Sri Ramakrishna of India (1836-
1886), we find many facts regarding the occurrences of physical variations as he changed his mental states. Many definite
physical changes of voluntary and involuntary functions of
his body took place at different times.

SUGGESTION

The development of will has a close connection with the
transference of thought. Human beings are gregarious. We
live in society; we are constantly influenced by one another;
and we give suggestions directly and indirectly to one another most of the time.

There are two types of suggestions. One is suggestion
through reason and logic, as we find when we read certain
books. In certain philosophies we follow the thinking process
and the thought current logically step by step. We appreciate
and absorb some of the ideas and ideals, and the suggestions
are taken rationally. Then there are suggestions which are
nonrational and nondeliberate. Take, for instance, the suggestions that are often given to us by our neighbors in the
course of our conversations. They may tell us stories of
ghosts or obsessions, and our conscious mind does not accept

[4] Swami Saradananda, *Sri Sri Ramakrishna Lilaprasanga*, Vol. II,
Sadhakabhava (Calcutta: Udbohan Office), chap. 14.

them but rather ridicules them. Yet the unconscious mind accepts the suggestion; and when we are in a lonely place or in a dark house, that idea arises and makes us afraid of something. This fear arises because the unconscious mind, at some time or other, nonrationally accepted certain suggestions and absorbed them. The unconscious mind is carrying out those suggestions. Often our well-meaning parents discourage us from doing certain things. "John, you and Mary should not go out in the dark night" is a negative idea, although John and Mary may not realize it. They unconsciously preserve that idea and in the darkness they feel a kind of nervousness. The suggestions concerning disease are deplorable. Nowadays, symptoms of certain diseases are discussed in newspapers, magazines, and other publications. Yet some of the symptoms are common to other diseases. For instance, take stomach disorders. Such ailments can result from hyperacidity and from nervousness; for when the nervous system is agitated and disturbed, it can cause a certain form of stomach disorder. Difficulties arise if something is eaten which is not suitable to the digestion of a person, or if he eats something when he is exhausted or emotionally upset. Sometimes symptoms may be due to an ulcer or malignant growth. When a person reads about symptoms of malignancy he thinks: "Perhaps I have a growth in my stomach." A fear obsesses him, and this very obsession disturbs the nervous system, creating a neurotic condition. We know of many such cases. Many of the psychoneuroses arise from false apprehension or fear, while the basis of the fear is nonrational and indirect suggestion.

Direct and indirect suggestion may be constructive or destructive, positive or negative. In a constructive suggestion we may receive the idea, in a direct logical process or even in direct conversation, that it is good to be loving. Perhaps in direct conversation some people have given us examples, and the unconscious mind conserves the idea that love conquers hatred. We do not have to read scriptures or go through all the teachings of logic to reach that conclusion. The mind accepts the suggestion. If I have a conviction that yes, love really conquers hatred, then when the occasion arises I shall try to practice it even unconsciously. On the other hand, as the result of negative or destructive suggestion there is hatred toward other races. Not long ago many of the people in this country associated a Chinese with laundries or restaurants; such a man was thought to be merely fit for laundry or restaurant work. People never realized that a Chinese could become a military genius, philosopher, industrialist, or banker. They thought that those qualities were the exclusive property of certain races and groups of people. Even now children are often given these ideas and actually believe they are true. Therefore, when they grow up these negative qualities are expressed. The disturbances between Jews and Christians are an instance. You will find negative ideas are often expressed directly or indirectly by parents; and the children imbibe those ideas and express them, too, even when they become adults, thinking that it is good to do something unkind to the other group—Christian or Jewish. These negative ideas are accepted, providing there is a certain amount of faith in them.

It will not be out of place to say here that Christian Science and New Thought groups often use the method of suggestion for treatment of their students. Whether scientific minds can accept the philosophy of these groups or not, it is true that in many cases this method has a certain ameliorating effect. Considerable influence from Hindu psychology is noticed in these groups. It is known to us that some of their leading members attended the lectures and classes of Swami Vivekananda in New York City during the nineties of the last century. We are also informed that Mrs. Eddy, the founder of Christian Science, acknowledged her indebtedness to the teachings of the *Bhagavad-Gita* in one of the early editions of *Science and Health*.[5] We do not imply that the leading personalities of the Christian Science and New Thought movements thoroughly and consistently adopted the Hindu philosophical and psychological systems. They only adapted certain ideas to their own plan of philosophy and practices.

HYPNOSIS

There are also methods of giving constructive and destructive deliberate suggestions such as hypnosis. Hypnosis is nothing but a conscious and deliberate suggestion given to a person who will accept and believe it. Both in ordinary suggestion as well as hypnotic suggestion there is one important factor—the attitude of the mind which receives the suggestion. Whether we call it deliberate suggestion or hypnosis does not make any difference. The mind must be in a mood to accept it, consciously or unconsciously. Sometimes we hear someone say that he can interest a person in an idea. A man may say: "You cannot influence me"; but in two minutes he is intrigued. He receives the suggestion because there is a belief in the possibility of his being influenced.

Freud and a number of the Western psychologists think that there must be a "transference" between a person who gives a suggestion and the person who receives it. Treatment by suggestion is extensively used by psychiatrists, and they believe that there is a transference between the doctor and the patient. Transference means a relationship between the person giving the suggestion and the one receiving it. It is often regarded as a transference of old, strong, deep-rooted,

[5] Mary Baker Eddy, *Science and Health*, (24th ed.; 1886), chap. 8, especially p. 259, cited by Swami Abhedananda, *Christian Science and Vedanta*, (7th ed.; San Francisco: Vedanta Ashrama, 1902), pp. 2-3.

and unexpressed emotion, although it might have been even
in the unconscious realm.

In spiritual life there must be more than just a relationship; there must be real obedience, devotion, and love on
the part of the student for the person who is giving the suggestion and training. Then it becomes dynamic and operative. Both Brown and McDougall differ from the Freudian
interpretation of libido in this respect: their opinion is that
the libidinal urge is not responsible for the receipt of suggestion, but it is the spirit of submission instead which allows
the mind to receive suggestion. Both of these great psychologists and many others believe that there is an inherent tendency in man to submit to others and that it is one of the
primitive urges of man. In fact, society cannot operate unless
there is such a tendency in human beings. We cannot learn
anything from our teachers, whether in college or in Sunday
school, unless we have the spirit of submission or receptivity.
Sometimes our young people resent the use of the word submission; they become offended lest their ego is being slighted.
But the fact remains that without the attitude of receiving
something from others we cannot learn anything in the
world, whether it is intellectual, moral, spiritual, or any
other type of knowledge. Therefore, there is a need of this
submissive spirit. Hindus say that suggestions become active
and dynamic only when there is a deep feeling or relationship between the person who gives suggestion and the person
who receives it. If there is no point of contact emotionally,
there will be no avenue of suggestion. The modern psychiatrist should observe this factor when he uses the method
of suggestion. Although mere release of old unexpressed
emotion and its transference to another person may bring
relief to an individual, we believe that it cannot help in
building up a personality.

Today, hypnotic practices have become more or less obsolete. Charcot, Janêt, and others used them to cure cases of neuroses or mental disturbances. Freud practiced this method in his earlier days until he developed psychoanalysis. Some psychiatrists still use hypnosis for the training of the memory process, but as a method of education it is not very good and should not be encouraged. The reason is clear. In hypnosis, the will of the person is kept in abeyance. He receives the suggestion from the hypnotizer and does not allow his own mind to function. The suggestion may be given to him: "You are shivering" or "You are sleeping," and it is allowed to go on to its maximum functioning at the cost of his own thinking or feeling. The person's mind is suspended from operation and the effect is deplorable. A man may say that he has cured a few obsessions or discovered some of the subconscious processes but, at the same time, he has greatly weakened the mind of the individual he has treated. It is true that once a person is hypnotized the effect remains for a long time. We are acquainted with some persons who have been hypnotized and know that the effect lasted for many years. Their nervous systems were weakened; their minds became passive and negative; and they were receptive to any suggestion or idea given to them. For instance, if someone said to any one of them: "You cannot do anything so how will you learn this?" or "You should not be allowed to go out alone," the individual would receive those negative ideas and feel that he was good for nothing. He would also think: "Perhaps what this man says is true; I have no possibility of doing something constructive or creative." We have known cases where such negative attitudes persisted for a long period of time because of the effect of hypnosis or similar suggestions. We also have observed that some of them often develop a kind of obstinate attitude and superiority complex later on to overcome the sense of inferiority. Some also try to show off by opposing anything that is discussed with a con-

E*

trary point of view. In fact, they reveal signs of extremely unusual tendencies which they never had until the hypnosis. The whole nervous system is shattered; therefore, hypnosis should not be encouraged even though it might appear that we can help the person to do good things. Temporary success should not encourage one to weaken permanently the will of any individual.

Coué, the French exponent of the theory of suggestion in psychotherapy, feels that in treatment by suggestion the client should not be allowed to use the will. He seems to feel that it creates conflict between suggestion and effort. However, the client fails to integrate his emotions, not because there is conflict between suggestion and will but rather because the will is incomplete. Brown, too, feels that the will must be allowed to function in its entirety. We also strongly advocate the complete functioning of the will in order to dissolve the conflict between emotions, primitive urges, and higher ideals and philosophy of life.

Hindu psychology is definitely against hypnotism, and although some of the teachers have developed elaborate methods of *bashi karan* hypnotism, or thought transference, they are always discouraged in this practice. As Swami Vivekananda says:

The so-called hypnotic suggestion can only act upon a weak mind. And until the operator, by means of fixed gaze or otherwise, has succeeded in putting the mind of the subject in a sort of passive, morbid condition, his suggestions never work.

·   ·   ·   ·   ·   ·   ·   ·   ·   ·

Every attempt at control which is not voluntary, not with the controller's own mind, is not only disastrous, but it defeats the end. The goal of each soul is freedom, mastery,—freedom from the slavery of matter and thought, mastery of external and internal nature. Instead of leading towards that, every will-current from another, in whatever form it comes, either as direct control of organs, or as forcing to control them while under a morbid condition, only rivets one link more to the already existing heavy chain of bondage of past thoughts, past superstitions. Therefore, beware how you allow yourselves to be acted upon by others. Beware how you unknowingly bring another to ruin. True, some succeed in doing good to many for a time, by giving a new trend to their propensities, but at the same time, they bring ruin to millions by the unconscious suggestions they throw around, rousing in men and women that morbid, passive, hypnotic condition which makes them almost soulless at last. Whosoever, therefore, asks any one to believe blindly, or drags people behind him by the controlling power of his superior will, does an injury to humanity, though he may not intend it.

Therefore, use your own minds, control body and mind yourselves, remember that until you are a diseased person, no extraneous will can work upon you . . . beware of everything that takes away your freedom. Know that it is dangerous, and avoid it by all the means in your power.[6]

Suspension of the voluntary functioning of the mind is always detrimental for the unification and integration of the will. Not only is hypnotic control positively harmful because the normal functioning of the mind is suspended, but it has also been found through experiment and study of drug addicts and habitual drunkards that they lose their will power, too; it is temporarily suspended while they remain under the influence of drugs or liquor. Then, as the habit of suspending the voluntary activities of the mind is formed, the will of such persons is gradually disintegrated, and they become almost powerless to complete an action at any given time. Consequently, they fail to succeed in anything which requires dynamic will.

One cannot be forced, however, to act under hypnotism if the action is against his moral susceptibilities. Some outstanding psychologists, such as William Brown, relate cases

6 *Works*, I, 172-73.

in which individuals have refused to act immorally in spite of their morbid condition. This proves that part of the mind (unconscious) remains in a way aware of what is going on, and the person must believe in the suggestions of the hypnotizer and be willing to accept them in order to be completely under their influence.

PERSONALITY

The problem of personality and development of will go together. A man cannot have a dynamic personality which affects the lives of others unless he has an integrated will. It is a peculiar fact that we cannot manage our own affairs and the affairs of our friends and relatives unless we have strong will. Let us not confuse strength with arrogance. People often think that in order to have personality they must have a kind of arrogance or that they must "bluff" the world. No, we cannot do it. Arrogance may have been effective in connection with a few persons. As Lincoln said: "You can fool some of the people all of the time, and all of the people some of the time, but you cannot fool all of the people all of the time." Arrogance is a limiting element. When we have egotism or arrogance, we separate ourselves from others. Personality makes us unified. A man who has personality appeals to all persons, while the arrogant person can control and use people for only a short time. Moreover, the activities of an arrogant man will ultimately create discord and confusion, while the activities of a man of real personality establish harmony and accord in useful production.

There is a marked difference between individuality and personality. Individuality is that particular quality which distinguishes one from the group. A man is short, and that quality of shortness distinguishes him from others. It may be physical individuality or it may be mental, intellectual, emotional, or some other type of individuality which separates a person from a group. There are some who confuse individuality with personality. Individuality, however, makes us limited while personality causes us to expand and gradually become universal.

We know that there are persons who possess something which attracts others. What is that attraction? Hindus tell us that our individual minds are part of the universal mind. As such, we are all basically connected with one another. Just as our individualized souls are part of the cosmic soul, so are our minds. Swami Vivekananda says:

> . . . There is a continuity of mind, as the Yogis call it. The mind is universal. Your mind, my mind, all these little minds, are fragments of that universal mind, little waves in the ocean; and on account of this continuity, we can convey our thoughts directly to one another.[7]

When a mind becomes active in its entirety by the development of will, it becomes connected with the cosmic existence. If there is a thought wave in a particular person, the vibrations of that thought will affect others. If a man of tremendous personality and purity lives in a cave in a remote corner of the globe and conceives a dynamic thought, that thought will influence the minds of the people in other parts of the world. Do we not believe that Jesus Christ was born about two thousand years ago, that He conceived a few dynamic thoughts and gave expression to them, and even today the vibrations are affecting us? Buddha expressed some powerful ideas about six centuries before Christ, and they are changing the people even now. We are surprised to note how the dynamic thoughts of Krishna, Buddha, Christ, and Sri Ramakrishna are affecting the present world. Sri Ramakrishna practiced religious harmony. His dynamic thoughts of

7 *Works,* II, 13.

harmony of religions are transforming people all over the world, and they are becoming liberal in their understanding and appreciation of other religions. Instead of denouncing religion they are accepting it. The writings of Romain Rolland, Professor Hocking, and others prove that the dynamic ideas of Sri Ramakrishna have a direct influence on the world. A recent book of Professor Hocking, *Living Religions and World Faith*, shows how the tendencies of the world are progressing. Professor Hocking is a devout Christian, rather than an agnostic or humanist, and when we read his book we fully realize how appreciative he is of other religions.

Our humble experiences with the religious leaders of Rhode Island, Massachusetts, and other states are extremely happy and cordial, to say the least. Our good friends Professor Brightman, Dean Marlatt, Dean Skinner, Dr. Claxton, Professor Johnson, Professor DeWolf, Dean Knudson, Professor Wach, Rabbi Braude, Rabbi Bilgray, and many others among the religious leaders and teachers are so friendly and cordial one would think that we had been brought up in the same environments. Many more names could be added to those already mentioned. This definitely proves that the whole atmosphere is changing radically among the deep thinkers and devotees. This has been the experience of many in our Order (the Swamis of the Ramakrishna Order) in the West. Not only in America but also in Europe the same has been found to be true in the favorable attitudes of many outstanding intellectualists, psychologists, rationalists, and scientific members of the universities.

The creating of personality does not lie in physical expressions but in the unification of mind. St. Francis of Assisi was not an attractive person so far as physical structure was concerned, nor was Abraham Lincoln. Yet we find that the thoughts of St. Francis and other such personalities influence others. Similarly, the ideas of Lincoln affect people deeply. As long as this country remains in existence, the ideal that was declared by Lincoln will be supported, honored, and appreciated. As long as the human mind has the power of thinking, the ideal of St. Francis of Assisi, and the thought of Swami Vivekananda will remain effective. A great scholar of India once expressed appreciation of Swami Vivekananda, saying that as long as the sun and the moon remained operative his contributions to Hindu culture would remain dynamic. This was declared by a man who was a scholar, not of a liberal school, but of a great orthodox Hindu school.

It is true that human magnetism lies in the development of the will and not in the culture of the body. When our emotions are wholly integrated, then alone the will becomes totally operative. Every child and every man in the world wants a dynamic, magnetic personality. Little do we understand that the personality cannot be developed until we unify the mind and integrate the emotions and the will. When a man's character is built with the development of his total mind, his thoughts, emotions, and will are integrated; the stamp of his character is found in each one of his actions. A man of personality is he who lives the ideal and not he who talks about it. There are many intellectual giants who beautifully explain philosophy, art, science, and religion. There are many persons who can give wonderful descriptions of religion and mysticism, yet those talks do not affect people because those ideals are not lived by the speakers. Their words may satisfy our intellect; but, on the other hand, the simple unsophisticated statements of a man of religious experience change the thought current and life of men, bringing out the inner perfection of innumerable persons. He does not utter a single word that he does not live, so his words usher in a new civilization. What makes the words of Jesus Christ so powerful is the life behind them. Such are the lives of Krishna, Buddha, and such other personalities, because their words were magnetized by the integrated will.

We have seen again and again how a few simple words of

great spiritual personalities changed the thought current of many disintegrated and disrupted men and women, who were transformed by the magnetic touch of such personalities. It was not because they could discuss theology, philosophy, or science but because they created an atmosphere of strong spiritual living. Transforming power was in their very integrated personalities. We remember a man who came to our monastery to dissuade his older brother from joining the Order. This man came in a drunken state; in fact, his life was anything but commendable. When he met one of the leading Swamis of this Order, who happened to be a man of high spiritual illumination, he was at first extremely antagonistic and ignoble to him. But that great spiritual personality, Swami Premananda—who was a disciple of Sri Ramakrishna—in an affectionate and loving manner addressed and tried to console him, saying that his brother would be allowed to return to his home if he chose to do so. Then the Swami gave him some refreshments to cool him off, as it was a very hot day. This man had never experienced such kind treatment. In spite of his abusive behavior, the Swami treated him as if he had known him all his life and when he was leaving requested him to come again to the monastery. Such loving treatment impressed the younger brother so much that he could not forget that magnetic personality. After that, he frequented the monastery and visited Swami Premananda. Instead of persuading his brother to leave, he himself finally remained there and became an ardent follower of the Swami. The influence of this spiritual leader transformed the man in an unbelievable way and made a noble personality—in fact, a religious leader—out of him. It is interesting to note that this transformed man not only lives an intensely religious life but has become a true servant of mankind, having built up a large hospital and relief center for the welfare of suffering humanity. The influence of the great Swami brought out what was best in him and made him a true servant of man and God.

We can cite a number of similar cases from the lives of Swami Vivekananda, Swami Brahmananda, and such others of our contemporary history. We do not have to cite the cases from the lives of Krishna, Buddha, Christ, and Sri Ramakrishna. Every historian knows how full of such instances are the lives of these incarnate spirits. The strength of such unified personalities lies in their religious experiences, nay, in their actual living of religion. Professor Allport very aptly says:

> Religion is the search for a value underlying ALL things, and as such is the most comprehensive of all the possible philosophies of life. A deeply moving religious experience is not readily forgotten, but is likely to remain as a focus of thought and desire.[8]

Therefore, when we want to influence others, when we want to change others, we must change our own lives by translating our ideals into dynamic will and consequent action. This is the secret of human magnetism. Swami Vivekananda says:

> ... The personality of the man is two-thirds, and his intellect, his words, are but one-third. It is the real man, the personality of the man, that runs through us. Our actions are but effects; actions must come when the man is there. ...
>
> The ideal of all education, all training, should be this man-making. But, instead of that, we are always trying to polish up the outside. ... The end and aim of all training is to make the man grow. The man who influences, who throws his magic, as it were, upon his fellow-beings, is a dynamo of power, and when that man is ready, he can do anything and everything he likes; that personality put upon anything will make it work.[9]

[8] Allport, *Personality, A Psychological Interpretation*, p. 226.
[9] *Works*, II, 15.

CHAPTER VI

Meditation

THE dynamic power of human personality cannot be developed without total integration of the mind. The three aspects of the human mind—cognition, emotion, and volition—must be unified in order to bring out all the latent possibilities in man. We already know that all glorious cultural activities throughout the history of the world have been directed and achieved by men and women of concentrated will power.

Hindu psychologists recognize that the will must be integrated completely and the mind must be made totally active in order to use all of its mental forces. They have even startled authorities of the positive sciences with their subjective training of the mind. The late Sir B. N. Seal, of Calcutta University, has shown how the positive sciences of the Hindus were developed by men and women with a thorough training in concentration of the mind.[1]

The practice of concentration is, no doubt, the kernel of religious evolution. Without the practice of concentration and meditation, no man can ever expect to reach the highest state of spiritual evolution. When we study the lives of the great Christian, Jewish, Hindu, Buddhist, and Mohammedan mystics, we fully realize that they reached the highest

[1] B. N. Seal, *The Positive Sciences of the Ancient Hindus* (London: Longmans, Green & Co., 1915).

spiritual consciousness through development of the power of concentration.

Apart from the religious and philosophical attainments of man through the practice of concentration, we also recognize its pragmatic value in the integration of the human mind and personality. So far as the dissolution of human conflicts is concerned, a man cannot successfully dissolve the conflicting emotions of the mind unless he has developed some power of concentration. It is clearly explained by the modern Western psychologists and psychiatrists, and also by the Hindu psychologists, that the human mind is an arena of conflicting urges and emotions. When a person with a great deal of emotional disturbance is analyzed by an expert psychiatrist, he may recognize the nature of the conflict. He may also understand that unless it is removed there is practically no hope for his mental peace and happiness. Apart from that, he may also realize that his functional ailments are produced by mental conflicts and frustration; yet the struggling person finds himself in an utterly helpless condition to overcome them in spite of self-analysis and psychoanalysis. We do know, however, that some persons are helped by these methods, but a permanent integration is not usually observed in them. The mind cannot be developed and strengthened by such methods alone, even when extreme restlessness is temporarily eliminated.

Many persons become attached to both pleasant and unpleasant experiences. They may doubt that they have attachment to the disagreeable incidents of life when it would seem natural to prefer to think of the pleasant things. Unfortunately, however, people do cling to apprehensions, fears, and other such unpleasant and disturbing feelings even though they know that their peace of mind is being destroyed. Their thoughts go on without any control whatsoever. Consequently, they cannot sleep; they become nervous; and then they get many functional ailments in brooding over apprehensions, fears, anxieties, and unpleasant incidents of life.

Professor William James realized the difficulty of emotional conflicts. He also recognized the utility of systematic training of the mind. According to him:

> The emotions and excitements due to usual . . . situations are the usual inciters of the will. But these act discontinuously; and in the intervals the shallower levels of life tend to close in and shut us off. Accordingly, the best practical knowers of the human soul have invented the thing known as methodical ascetic discipline to keep the deeper levels constantly in reach. It is, I believe, admitted that the disciples of asceticism can reach very high levels of freedom and power of will.[2]

Hindus realize the utility of the practice of concentration. So far as our experience goes with the disturbed conditions of the human mind, we are entirely convinced that without the practice of concentration one cannot expect to gather the mental forces which are already scattered and dissipated by emotional urges and conflicts. Steady practice of concentration relaxes the mind; the restless thoughts become single and one-pointed; and then the nervous system becomes relaxed so that a person can get sleep and rest. Swami Vivekananda says: "Never say any man is hopeless, because he only represents a character, a bundle of habits, which can be checked by new and better ones."[3]

Indian psychologists have developed a science of this concentration. Patanjali, the father of *Raja Yoga* (applied psychology), gives us an elaborate treatment of the science of concentration. He gives eight steps to the perfect state of concentration (superconsciousness): *yama* (mental control),

---

[2] William James, " The Energies of Man." *Memories and Studies* (London: Longmans, 1911), p. 251.
[3] *Works*, I, 208.

niyama (physical regulation and special mental training), *asana* (posture), *pranayama* (breathing exercises), *pratyahara* (withdrawal of mind from sense objects), *dharana* (concentration), *dhyana* (meditation), and *samadhi* (superconsciousness). These are the gradual steps to be followed in order to reach the goal. It was recognized by James that "the most venerable ascetic system, and the one whose results have the most voluminous experimental corroboration, is undoubtedly the Yoga system in Hindustan."[4] According to Patanjali, a man must practice concentration systematically by focusing the mind on one object in order to unify his mental forces.[5] In the beginning, of course, it may take a little time to achieve the desired power of concentration, as the mind has already been scattered. Swami Brahmananda says:

> By regular practice it [the mind] can be quieted and brought under restraint. . . . In the beginning meditation proves very difficult and dry. But if you persist, as in the taking of a medicine, you will find in it a perennial source of joy, pure and unalloyed.[6]

It is also said in the *Bhagavad-Gita* that the mind is restless, no doubt, and hard to subdue. But it can be brought under control by constant practice, and by the exercise of dispassion.[7]

Ancient and modern Indian psychologists agree that even though the practice of concentration is difficult, it can be achieved by everyone through systematic practices. In the beginning we are to take certain concrete objects for the purpose of concentration. As our minds are attracted by the objective world, our sense organs and instruments are also

[4] James, *Memories and Studies*, p. 251.
[5] The system of Patanjali is based on certain conceptions in the Sankhya system of Hindu thought.
[6] *Spiritual Teachings of Swami Brahmananda* (2nd ed.; Mylapore, Madras: Sri Ramakrishna Math, 1933), p. 100.
[7] *Srimad-Bhagavad-Gita* VI:35.

constituted in such a way as to be constantly outgoing.[8] Therefore, the mind is being constantly supplied with new sensations and experiences, and it remains jumpy and extremely restless because of the influx of new materials and subsequent mental reactions.[9] Moreover, we have already accumulated the residuals of our past experiences in the subconscious region. They are constantly operative in the subconscious and also try to force themselves up to the conscious plane. The result is that the mind behaves like a monkey, as Swami Vivekananda so beautifully illustrated in his *Raja Yoga*.[10]

The nervous system is also extremely agitated because of restless states of the mind. Until it attains higher states of consciousness, the mind functions almost entirely through the nervous system. When the nervous system is affected, the mind is also affected, and vice versa. So the Hindu psychologists prescribe two steps preliminary to mental concentration—*yama* (ethical observation and mental control) and *niyama* (physical cleansing and dietetic restrictions etc. and certain mental training).[11] Non-killing, truthfulness, non-stealing, continence, internal and external purification, contentment, and self-control constitute *yama* and *niyama*.[12] In the beginning, one should try to cleanse the mind and body through proper purificatory processes. The nervous system can be made stronger by certain simple dietetic regulations. We all know that when we take a stimulant or drug, our systems are either overstimulated or made dull. On the other hand, when we take soothing, nutritious, and wholesome food or liquids, the nervous system and the whole body remain quiet. A certain amount of simple regulation about

[8] *Katha Upanishad* 4:1.
[9] *Gita* II:62-68.
[10] *Works*, I, 174.
[11] *Ibid.*, 137.
[12] *Ibid.*, 260-61.

food and drink is helpful in the beginning of the practice of concentration, so that the mind and nervous system may not be overstimulated and excited or deadened and made dull. The mental cleansing is even more important than the physical cleansing. Unfortunately, experience has demonstrated that when physical improvement is overemphasized, man often neglects mental health and, above all, spiritual development. As a result, the *Hatha Yogis* developed the culture of physical power as well as some of the extraordinary psychic and occult powers; and, unfortunately, many of them neglected and ignored spiritual development. We also observe in many groups in America, and in other places, that when people become extremely interested in physical development they often become faddists at the cost of real mental health and spiritual growth. Swami Vivekananda was in favor of the middle path with just the simple observation of physical health.[13]

Professor James seemed to be convinced that certain mental and physical exercises are useful for the total development of the mind. He describes a case in "The Energies of Man" and tells that a friend of his went through certain Hindu *yoga* disciplines which had a wonderful effect.[14]

Inner cleansing is of vital importance so far as mental integration and the practice of concentration is concerned. We know that the human mind becomes extremely disturbed and agitated by some of the primitive urges and secondary emotions such as ambition, anger, hatred, jealousy, and envy. We also know, through our own observation and experience, that as long as the tendencies of the inordinate emotions are very strong the mind will remain always restless. Patanjali, in his first chapter of Aphorisms on *Raja Yoga*, prescribes the cultivation of satisfaction and contentment and other

[13] *Ibid.,* 136.
[14] James, *Memories and Studies,* p. 253.

such qualities. He also suggests that when a person expresses an extreme form of suspicion, jealousy, or hatred he should be advised to cultivate the opposite tendencies deliberately. Nothing spoils human peace and happiness more thoroughly than such ill-directed emotions. We know from the study of different cases that human lives have been completely ruined by suspicion, hatred, jealousy, anger, and extreme ambition. Patanjali advocates that a man who has these tendencies, regardless of the justice of his cause, should be advised aggressively to cultivate friendliness, generosity, and affection toward the individuals against whom he has ill feelings. It may be painful and disagreeable sometimes; yet one must try, at least subjectively, to create constructive tendencies, for they help one to curb the restlessness of the mind.

As we struggle to overcome the disturbing conditions of the mind due to disappointment, frustration, or conflict, we also must cultivate positively the power of concentration and meditation. It is a peculiar situation in which most people find themselves. It is almost like a vicious circle. A man cannot have the proper power of concentration unless he has, to some extent, dissolved the conflicting urges and the sense of frustration. On the other hand, he cannot overcome these disturbing elements of the mind unless he tries to achieve the power of concentration. So one should deliberately try to combine the process of overcoming conflicts and frustrations with the positive method of cultivating opposite and higher constructive emotions together with the steady practice of meditation.

It is desirable that one should try to relax the body when one practices concentration. The nervous systems of most people are so tense that even when they try to go to sleep they cannot rest properly. Physical relaxation is extremely helpful for mental repose, so the Hindu psychologists advise one to sit in a relaxed position (*asana*) and let the whole neuromuscular system loosen up. This gradually helps one to relax the entire nervous system at will. Although it may seem unlikely, experience reveals that this practice performed in the morning and evening helps the relaxation of the neuromuscular system at other times. It is also observed that, when certain exciting causes appear, one can willfully relax the neuromuscular system and remove the nerve tension and consequent mental disturbances. We do not mean here that the mind is the product of the nervous system; but we cannot help recognizing that, for the time being, the mind is greatly dependent on the nature of the functioning of the nervous system. There comes a time in the course of mental development, however, when the mind itself can wholly control the nervous system.

Rhythmical breathing (*pranayama*) is also found to be efficacious. When a person practices it, the nervous system becomes quiet and the mind becomes calm. Some of the psychologists of India, particularly the *Raja Yogis* and *Hatha Yogis*, advocate a certain type of breathing exercise for the practice of concentration, although one should be judicious and careful in taking up certain vigorous practices in breathing. Some of the vigorous *pranayama* practices should be followed only under the direction of a good and expert teacher and should also be accompanied with certain dietetic regulations and rigorous mental discipline. Stimulating and deadening food and drink should be strictly avoided. Otherwise, there is danger of creating disturbances both in the nervous system and in the mind. However, simple rhythmical breathing of short duration is found to be helpful in many cases. We want definitely to make it clear that, although simple or vigorous breathing exercises are helpful for relaxation, they are not absolutely necessary for the practice of concentration.

After practicing relaxation for a few minutes, one should take a symbol or personal aspect of God on which to focus

the mind. In the practice of concentration, one should eliminate all thoughts except that of the particular symbol or
aspect of God. One should focus the entire mind on that
particular being or object of concentration and hold it before
the mind as much as possible. In the beginning, one will
observe that the mind runs away to previous thoughts and to
objects of the senses which were previously experienced. One
should try to withdraw the mind from these objects and
thoughts (*pratyahara*). It is observed that, unfortunately,
unpleasant and disagreeable experiences come to the surface
of the mind usually at that time. That is the very reason
Jesus, the Christ, says:

> If therefore thou art offering thy gift at the altar, and there
> rememberest that thy brother hath aught against thee, leave there
> thy gift before the altar, and go thy way, first be reconciled to
> thy brother, and then come and offer thy gift.[15]

Patanjali and other great psychologists of India always
emphasize that one should cultivate a peaceful state of mind
by adopting a sound philosophy of life. As we said previously,
one should deliberately create a pleasant and friendly atmosphere about one's self. One must try to overcome hatred,
envy, jealousy, and other such negative feelings, in order to
have a peaceful state of mind. Sound ethical principles are
absolutely necessary. As the mind becomes quiet and relaxed,
one can succeed in concentrating it on the desired object
(*Ishta*). But the mind must be one-pointed (*dharana*).

One should not be discouraged and give up the practice of
concentration when it is difficult to hold the mind on God
for more than a few seconds. In the course of practice for a
period of months, one can gain power to hold continuously
the thought of the particular aspect or desired symbol of
God. One should ignore the restlessness of the mind in the

[15] Matt. 5:23-24.

beginning. It is but natural that the mind will be considerably agitated during the first period of the practice of concentration, as it is still full of subconscious restless tendencies, conflicts, and disturbances. But experience proves that
the mind becomes steady and peaceful within a short time.
Progress depends upon the intensity of practice.[16]

The result of the practice of concentration and meditation
will depend upon the choice of the object. Sometimes, we
are amused to note that people advocate focusing the mind
on any object whatsoever in order to develop spiritually.
Patanjali describes elaborately in *Raja Yoga* the various types
of objects of concentration that are taken up by the pupil for
different reasons. If we concentrate the mind on material
particles or material entities, we can gain the power of concentration, no doubt; yet the result will be quite different
from what we will get in concentrating on an aspect of God.
Man can develop occult, psychic, and other extraordinary
mental powers like levitation, suspension of breath, emanation of light, thought reading, or thought transference.[17]
Control of some of the laws of nature can be developed
through concentration on different material objects and
other subtle objects. These types of concentration may satisfy
the curiosity of certain individuals and may also give some
kind of power over nature and people; yet, ultimately, they
do not help the integration of the total personality of a man.
A few years ago, a man from India, Khoda Box, demonstrated the power of not being burnt in the presence of the
Medical Association in London. It was, no doubt, an amazing
and interesting display. We know personally some individuals
in India who have extraordinary powers which seem to
overcome what we call "laws of nature." But we frankly
admit that they have not succeeded in the integration of

[16] *Yoga Aphorisms of Patanjali* I:21-22.
[17] *Ibid.*, chap. III.

their personalities, in spite of this unusual display of power. They cannot be regarded as spiritual persons. We are interested, primarily, in mental development and spiritual evolution and not in the control of the laws of nature or display of extraordinary psychic or occult powers.

The *Raja Yogis*, the great Indian psychologists, warn people against the display of such powers. Buddha turned out one of his followers who unconsciously developed some extraordinary powers which are known commonly as miracles. Many persons in certain Christian groups become enthusiastic about these miracles because Jesus performed them. But they do not realize that a man of His type had the power to remain unaffected by them as He was established in God-consciousness. He says: "An evil and adulterous generation seeketh after a sign. . . ."[18] Other Hindu authorities also tell us that extraordinary powers (*siddhis*) are obstacles to higher mental and spiritual evolution. Patanjali describes the methods of developing these powers and then warns that a sincere seeker of truth must not indulge in such practices.[19] Sri Ramakrishna emphatically discourages the manifestation of these extraordinary occult and psychic powers. He definitely says that a man cannot evolve spirtually as long as his mind dwells upon them; moreover, one becomes degraded in the course of the expression of these powers. He also says:

Visit not the miracle mongers and the exhibitors of occult powers. These men are stragglers from the path of truth. Their minds have become entangled in the meshes of psychic powers which come in the way of the pilgrim to Brahman [Absolute].[20]

His great disciples also discouraged every one of us from having any interest in such practices. We are entirely con-

[18] Matt. 12:39.
[19] *Yoga Aphorisms of Patanjali*, chap. III.
[20] *Sayings of Sri Ramakrishna* (Mylapore, Madras: Sri Ramakrishna Math, 1925), chap. XXXVI:696.

vinced that one must be extremely careful in his choice of
the object of concentration.

When concentration is very deep and the mind does not
waver but remains focused on the object of thought, that is
meditation (*dhyana*). According to Hindu psychologists,
meditation is not merely a nice thought, a poetic flight, or
loose fancies of even pleasant experiences; it is the depth of
concentration in which the mind flows continuously to an
object without any cessation as "oil poured from one vessel
to another." It is not a succession of many thoughts of the
same object. The mind must not waver whatsoever. So a man
is really meditating when his mind is freed from all other
thoughts and is wholly focused on the object of his concentration.

Methods in the practice of concentration, however, are
different according to various types of mind. There are some
psychologists who advocate the practice of emptying the
mind entirely for the time being. They advise the student to
make the mind a vacuum by eliminating or controlling all
thoughts that try to arise. There is, however, a danger in this
form of practice in the beginning. When one is not strong
enough mentally, one may enter into a negative passive state,
and then in that state the subconscious urges can become
operative as all controls and censorships are withdrawn.
Some of the modern groups say that they can get the voice
and direction of God by keeping the mind a vacuum. It is
rather risky to depend on such experiences as being valid.
Weaker persons (as most beginners are) have unintegrated
minds that are likely to contain bubbles of old residuals of
past experiences in the subconscious region, and these may
erroneously be regarded as the guidance or voice of God.
This false "guidance" may console us and give us a kind of
self-satisfaction, yet it does not help us to integrate and
strengthen the mind and to have higher spiritual evolution.

We do not advocate that anyone take up this method in the early stages of the practice of concentration unless he has a proper guide. It might be self-deceptive and extremely disappointing in the long run. The later Buddhistic philosophers, religious teachers, and psychologists understood the limitation of this form of meditation. Consequently, they advocated the adoption of the personal aspect of Buddha as the object of concentration, meditation, worship, adoration, and love. They also began to use symbols and forms and developed a science of symbology. However, we admit that there are some highly intellectual persons in every age who can take up this method even in the beginning and achieve great success.

The majority of the people should adopt a personal aspect of God as the object of meditation. It is desirable to take an aspect that is suitable to the temperament and background of the individual. If a devout Christian wants to practice concentration, he should take Jesus or the Madonna as his ideal and concentrate the mind on one or the other. With a Hindu background, a person can take any of the Incarnations who are loved by the Hindus. If one is of Jewish tradition, he should take an aspect of God that is suitable to him according to his tradition and background. There are some persons who feel that they are unable to adopt a bodily aspect of God for their concentration. Sometimes, philosophically speaking, they find it difficult to accept God as a person with form. There are people all over the world who feel it almost objectionable to their sense of dignity to associate the Infinite, the Absolute, with a body and form. From a rational point of view, we do not find any objection in taking a physical aspect of God. It is possible to have a conception of the Absolute as attributeless and beyond time-space relationship, but the bodily aspect of God is the highest understanding of the Impersonal by the human mind. That is to say, when the human mind tries to understand God, it necessarily thinks of Him in terms of its experiences. At present, our minds are in a state in which we cannot conceive or think of a thing that has no name, form, and attributes and that has no time-space relationship. We are in the habit of thinking of things that have name, form, and qualities that are existing in time and space. It is almost impossible to fix the mind, which is extremely restless at first, on something which cannot even be conceived by the mind. To illustrate this point, let us think of electricity. You cannot teach the nature of electricity to a child or to an average man without pointing to its manifestation in the form of light, heat, or motion. A man understands electricity when he sees its power revealed in the lamp, stove, or engine. He does not understand abstract electricity; therefore, if he has to concentrate his mind on it, he must think of it in its manifested state as light, heat, or motion. Similarly, if we are to concentrate on God, the Absolute, we can do it more easily when we focus the mind on His manifested state in a visible God, an Incarnation, or a symbol—*sakar* and *saguna* (with form and attributes).

One should be particular in the understanding of the symbol in order to use it as an object of concentration. It must signify the universal qualities of God; otherwise, it will not give us the desired spiritual realization. It may, however, give the power of concentration and thereby develop occult or psychic powers and other extraordinary phenomena.

It is convenient to focus the mind on a visible and bodily aspect of God or an Incarnation and meditate on Him, if we try to direct our emotions to Him. It is easy and natural for a man to think of a person whom he loves. A mother does not need to make an effort to think of her child; a husband or wife does not have to struggle to think of the wife or husband; a person does not need to discipline himself to think of his friend, because there is an emotional pull toward the friend, as there is toward one's own child, husband, or wife. That is the very reason that Patanjali and other Hindu psychologists, as well as great Christian, Buddhist, Jewish, and other mystics advocate the cultivation of love for a visible personal aspect of God.

One can also take God with qualities and attributes yet not with bodily form (*saguna* and *nirakara*). There are many persons in India and the West who prefer a personal aspect of God yet they do not care to think of Him with a physical form. They believe that God has attributes and qualities like "consciousness" and "love" without form. We can specially mention the personalistic schools of philosophy in America and Europe, of which the late Professor Bowne, Professor Brightman, Professor Hocking, and others are strong advocates, though they may differ in their interpretation of qualities and attributes. According to Professor Brightman: "God is a Person supremely conscious, supremely valuable, and supremely creative, yet limited both by the free choices of other persons and by restrictions within his own nature."[21]

We should make it clear that the Hindu view of the Impersonal God does not mean that God is not a conscious Being. According to the Impersonalists or Absolutists of Hindu schools, God is without attributes and form (*nirguna* and *nirakara*), invisible and beyond the categories of mind— Existence, Consciousness, and Bliss-Absolute (*Satchidananda*). He is pure Consciousness Itself, Self-conscious, and Self-luminous. "*Yat Vai Tat Sukham Raso Vai Saha, Rasam Hyevayam Labdhwanandi Bhavati.*" "That One who is Self-

[21] Edgar S. Brightman, *The Problem of God* (New York: The Abingdon Press, 1930), p. 113. For a full treatment of the idea of God see *The Problem of God*, chap. VI, and *A Philosophy of Religion* (New York: Prentice-Hall, Inc., 1940), chaps. V-X.

made is verily the joy. Having attained this joy, man becomes blessed."[22] He is beyond empirical consciousness as understood by the finite mind and He is beyond mind and speech. "*Avam Manasah Gocharam.*" "There goes neither I, nor speech, nor mind."[23] "This Atman can never be reached by speech, nor even by mind."[24] Sri Sankaracharya and other non-dualists explain that as It is Absolute Existence, Consciousness, and Bliss; It is beyond human expression and interpretation. Sri Ramakrishna says: "The Absolute and Unconditioned cannot be stated in terms of the Relative, the Conditioned. The Infinite cannot be expressed in terms of the Finite."[25] And Swami Vivekananda says: "The Personal God is the highest reading that can be attained to, of that Impersonal, by the human intellect."[26] Sri Ramakrishna harmonizes the three apparent distinct attitudes and interpretations of God as the different aspects of the same reality: (1) bodily and visible with attributes; (2) invisible yet with qualities and attributes (as the Personalists of America, some Hindus and Mohammedans, and others believe); (3) invisible and beyond qualities and attributes.[27] These aspects of the Reality can be realized by the devotees and seekers of truth in evolutionary stages through spiritual discipline.

It is important to remember that the development of power through concentration and meditation and consequent spiritual evolution depends greatly on the choice of the ideal or *Ishta.* A teacher of high spiritual attainment can detect the spiritual requirements and inherent tendencies of the student and help him in the choice of an object for meditation. Hindu psychologists and spiritual teachers em-

[22] *Taittiriya Upanishad,* Vol. VII, *Brahmananda Valli.*
[23] *Kena Upanishad* 1:3.
[24] *Katha Upanishad* 6:12.
[25] *Gospel of Sri Ramakrishna* (5th ed.; Mylapore, Madras: Sri Ramakrishna Math, 1930), I, 92.
[26] *Works,* I, 376.
[27] *Gospel,* I, 98.

F

phasize greatly the individual choice of an ideal, as no two minds are alike; nor can two minds have identical loving relationships, and attitudes toward God, even though they have been brought up in the same tradition and background. It has been found through experience that different members of the same family have loving devotion to different aspects of God and live together in harmony in spite of the divergence. Hindu psychologists, therefore, emphasize that instructions should be given individually regarding the object of meditation.

In the vast majority of cases of divine relationship, people have to cultivate attraction for God by creating a thought of Him. External and internal worship and the remembrance of the incidents in the lives of divine personalities are chosen to stimulate thoughts of God. The repetition of the name of God is helpful in the practice of meditation. The Hindus have developed a science of the name of God (*mantra vidya*), as well as a science of worship. A volume could be written on the technique of *mantra* alone. However, it may be said here that different aspects of God are represented by special names. The aspects, names, and forms are inseparable. "His manifesting word is Om." "The repetition of this (Om) and meditating on its meaning is the way."[28] When a devotee repeats a particular name of God, that aspect becomes a dominant factor in his life. The more he repeats the name of God which is suitable for him, the more he realizes the presence of God. This repetition definitely establishes a loving relationship between God and the devotee. It is observed historically that many devotees have reached higher states of mental development and integration and also spiritual evolution through repetition of the name of God. It will not be out of place to repeat here that special instructions are

[28] *Yoga Aphorisms of Patanjali* I:27-28, and *Works*, I, 217-20.

needed in the choice of a particular name of God associated
with the particular aspect.

These processes become very effective in establishing
higher emotional relationship with God. Once it is established, concentration and meditation become spontaneous
and enjoyable. One does not then need to struggle to withdraw the mind from the objective sense world. The mind
naturally flows to God. Swami Brahmananda says:

Remember Him when you eat, when you sit or when you lie
down. If you practice in this way, you will find that when you sit
down to meditate your mind will naturally become absorbed in
God. As your mind becomes absorbed in its meditation, a foun-
tain of joy will spring forth from within.[29]

All the religious teachers, the great men of God, admit that
there is an inseparable connection between the individual
soul and "over soul" or God. Yet because our minds are so
preoccupied by the objective experiences of the world and
have divergent interests and conflicts, it is not so easy and
natural for most people to feel the attraction for God. Consequently, the above practices become extremely helpful in
calming the mind, unifying the emotions, and, ultimately, in
establishing a person in meditation.

There are also methods for the gradual training of individuals who have no inclination to think of a personal God. The
great scientific minds or rationalistic thinkers find it difficult
to adopt a personality on which to concentrate. As Sir Arthur
Keith says:

I felt then as I do now that "Lord" is a dangerous word too apt
to assume a human shape, and this shape it did assume in the
minds of my critics. My fellow contributors are happier in their
choice; they speak of "an immortal essence," "a pervading spir-

[29] The Eternal Companion (Hollywood: Vedanta Society of Southern California, 1944), pp. 143-44.

itual force," "a principle of guiding good," "a great first cause."
... The poet may be justified in speaking of the universe as God's
visible garment, but such a God or Creator is one to which
science applies an altogether different nomenclature.[30]

There are many such persons who find it difficult to take a
personal aspect of God, whether with form or without form,
or "Lord, which is an unhappy one," according to Sir
Arthur. They have to adopt the impersonal aspect of God,
although that Impersonal Being is beyond the categories of
the human mind for the time being. That is the very reason
Swami Vivekananda strongly advised the use of a symbol or
substitute for the Impersonal.[31] Unfortunately, as we explained, our human minds cannot all at once adapt themselves to an object of meditation which has no quality or
attribute or name and form. Although these persons find it
"unhappy" and difficult to accept intellectually a visible
aspect of God, their minds are not trained enough to go
beyond the time-space relationship and the conditions of
name and form. The Unconditioned Being, the Absolute,
cannot be the object of thought and meditation in their
present state of development. As we practice concentration,
we are still cultivating the thought. Therefore, Hindu psychologists advocate strongly the use of symbols, such as light
or universal sound, to signify the universal qualities of the
Impersonal. Sri Ramakrishna says: "The key to the realization of the Absolute is with the Divine Person alone, the
Saguna Brahman of the *Upanishads*, the Personal God of
Devotees."[32] When a person is trained to meditate on the
personal aspect of God, he can transcend the limitations of
time, space, and causation and reach the Impersonal; but it is

[30] Clifton Fadiman (ed.). *I Believe* (New York: Simon and Schuster, 1939),
p. 379.
[31] *Works*, III, 59.
[32] *Gospel of Sri Ramakrishna*, I, 105.

well-nigh impossible for an average person to focus his mind on the Impersonal Being, the Absolute, in the beginning of the practice of concentration and meditation. Many persons may be well developed intellectually yet, unfortunately, emotionally they are on the lower step of the ladder. Thus there is a great deal of confusion in their thinking as well as in their practice of meditation. Sometimes we find that such people become dissatisfied with meditation as they can neither accept a personal God as an ideal nor reach the Impersonal. They seem to be neither "fish nor fowl." The solution is for them to realize that, although the Impersonal may be their ultimate object of meditation, yet, because of the way they are constituted for the time being, they cannot help but take a visible aspect of God or symbol of the Impersonal. In course of time, when they inwardly evolve, they will find that they can then go beyond the limitations of mind to the Absolute.

Some persons who seem outwardly intellectual are internally very emotional. Sometimes their emotional life seems frustrated and dissatisfied. Meditation on the Impersonal would not be helpful to them. They should be convinced rationally that for psychological reasons and for the unification of their emotions they ought to direct their minds to a personal aspect of God. When they achieve stability through that method, the emotional conflicts are dissolved, the sense of frustration loses its hold over the mind, and there is great inward satisfaction. As a result, that individual gradually becomes ready for meditation on the Impersonal. The religious history of the world proves to us definitely that there have been persons who started their spiritual practices and concentration and meditation with the personal aspect of God and, as they evolved, they gradually reached the Impersonal. Swami Brahmananda says:

It is best to start from Dualism. If you proceed a little along
this path, you will find that you are naturally led to Non-dualism.
To see God outside ourselves is a right path. Afterwards you
will be able to see God within yourself. This is the highest form
of meditation.[33]

There are innumerable variations in the mental constitution and inherent tendencies of people; so, as we have seen,
details in the methods of the practice of concentration and
meditation will be different. That is the very reason that
Swami Brahmananda definitely advocates in his *Spiritual
Teachings* that individual instruction—or what the Hindus
technically call initiation—is absolutely necessary in India.
All Indian books on higher psychology and spiritual instructions emphasize this. Says Swami Brahmananda:

Initiation is necessary because it helps concentration. When
you are initiated you are shown the object upon which the mind
is to be concentrated. You cannot let your mind waver from one
thing to another. If you are not initiated, you have no particular
object to concentrate upon. . . . A grim restlessness is the result.
This is most harmful to an aspirant. Until this state is overcome
and replaced by a peaceful attitude of mind, spiritual realization
will ever remain a distant prospect.[34]

However, one can take up the practice of concentration and
meditation individually until he meets a person who can
give definite instructions. We are giving a few general ideas
here for this purpose.

The best time for practice is the conjunction of day and
night—that is, early in the morning or early in the evening.
This may not always be practical for many Western people
as their routine of life is full of activity. It will be more convenient for them to practice meditation immediately after
awaking from sleep, as that is the time the mind generally

[33] *Spiritual Teachings of Swami Brahmananda*, p. 154.
[34] *Ibid.*, p. 102.

remains quiet. One can practice in the early part of the evening or just before retiring. Midday is also considered a good period for meditation.

One should first freshen one's self before sitting for meditation. Then a quiet corner and a special seat should be selected, if possible, for everyday practice. Regularity in the practice of meditation is of vital importance. When one practices regularly at a certain hour each day, it becomes a habit for the mind to be peaceful, particularly at that time. One can begin with ten-minute periods and gradually and steadily increase the duration. It should be remembered that an aspirant must not be overenthusiastic and suddenly start long periods of practice or sit for varying and irregular lengths of time. People often get an unfavorable reaction when they become overzealous for a few days, and they give up the practice of concentration and meditation altogether. Irregularity both in time and in duration is an obstacle for the unification of mental life.

The aspirant should relax the whole body at first and sit erect, keeping the upper part of the body and the spinal column straight. It is not so essential to sit in a cross-legged position, which strains the joints, muscles, and ligaments. Proper posture is important, yet one must not make one's self uncomfortable so that the mind is distracted and disturbed. It should always be remembered that meditation is primarily connected with the mind. Posture and breathing exercises are only meant to help the mind become quiet.

After relaxing the body and sitting in a proper position, one should take an aspect or symbol of God, as we previously discussed, and focus the mind on that, and that alone. The form or symbol should be visualized inside of one's self. It is true that some persons find it convenient to visualize the object of concentration outside, but it is better to try to think of the ideal as being within. Then as consciousness of the inner ideal develops, one becomes aware of it outside and in other people. In the beginning it is difficult to visualize the ideal within as we are generally in the habit of experiencing things objectively. It is good to keep a picture of the particular aspect of God or a symbol of God in the room or rooms which the aspirant frequents. The visual impression of the ideal creates a tendency toward further visualization. This is extremely helpful for the practice of concentration as it creates a conscious and unconscious thought form of the ideal. It is also helpful for concentration to repeat the name of God, especially the name of that aspect on which one meditates. Swami Brahmananda says:

When you sit in meditation, first think of a blissful divine form. This will have a soothing effect upon your nerves. Otherwise meditation will become dry and tedious. Think of the form of your Chosen Ideal, smiling and full of joy.[35]

We would like to strike a note of warning so that the aspirant may not become discouraged when he finds it difficult to visualize the ideal or feel the presence of God. Sometimes a person thinks that perhaps another symbol would be better for concentration than the one already chosen. However, the object should not be changed for any other until the person is thoroughly established in it and is ready to make the change. This does not necessarily make one narrow or bigoted; the aspirant should remember that other objects and symbols are expressions of the same God or Absolute, even though a particular aspect is suitable for the higher development of an individual.

It takes six months to a year to feel the effect of steady practice in the earlier days of psychological training, as the thought forms have to be changed. It has been noticed that many of the residuals of past experiences remain in the sub-

[35] *The Eternal Companion*, p. 127.

conscious region and they come to the surface and disturb the mind. It is also observed that some of the subtle impressions from other minds, outside influences, and negative thought currents often affect a person while he is struggling to meditate. One must not become discouraged by any of these influences nor should one consider whether or not he is progressing. He must continue the practice steadily for some time. Then he can feel the effect of meditation in mental and physical relaxation, restfulness, and also in the quality of the meditation itself. It is observed that higher ethical and spiritual qualities gradually become manifest in the person who practices concentration and meditation. Swami Brahmananda's advice to aspirants is:

Therefore perform a little meditation every day, and never fail to do it. The nature of the mind is to run away like a restless boy. Drag it back whenever it seeks to go out, and set it to meditating on God. If you can continue this struggle for two or three years, you will find in you a joy unspeakable . . .[36]

[36] *Spiritual Teachings of Swami Brahmananda*, p. 100.

F *

CHAPTER VII

Effect of Meditation

THERE are critics of the practice of concentration and meditation among the religious groups as well as among those who are outside the field of religion. Some of the religious people seem to think that it makes one passive and negative. They are almost afraid of even the name of meditation, thinking that it will take initiative away from their minds and make them vague or negative. They, no doubt, advocate doing good to others through social service and philanthropic work; yet in a peculiar way, they are critical of and antagonistic to the practice of meditation. We often hear it said that Occidental people should not follow the so-called Oriental practice of meditation because it will make them other-worldly and passive. The implication is that they are aggressive, dynamic, and intellectual and, therefore, not suited to habits of contemplation. Some persons even go to the extent of saying that the Occidental mind is fitted only for scientific methods of observation and experiment, or, in other words, that the people of the West are best suited to the study of the objective world in an objective sense.

Professor Jung was appreciative of the effect of the practice of concentration and meditation in Oriental countries like India and China, yet it was his opinion that the methods adopted in the Oriental countries could not be adapted to Occidental types of mind. He seemed to feel that Occidental people should develop a technique of their own. Such an opinion cannot be justified by the study of the lives and teachings of Oriental and Occidental mystics. St. Teresa of Avila says:

If you had asked me about meditation, I could have instructed you and advised anyone to practice it even though they do not possess the virtues, for this is the first step to obtain them all; it is vital for all Christians to begin this practice.[1]

St. Teresa, St. Ignatius, and others emphasized the utility of the practice of contemplation, concentration, and meditation; and none of them wearied of advising their followers to take up these methods. We do not find any fundamental differences between their systems of practice and those advocated by the Hindu teachers. What difference we find is between devotional and intellectual types of mentality rather than between Oriental and Occidental minds. This difference is observed even within the same group, either Oriental or Occidental, where there are various mental types, as we shall see in the chapter on "Methods of Superconscious Experience."

The critics among the nonreligious groups naturally disregard the practice of meditation, not because they know anything about its technique and its real effect, but because in their eyes it is a kind of mysterious habit as it is practiced by Oriental people. The tendency to regard meditation as mystifying is, we are afraid, colored by the achievements of Western science and its application to everyday life. The objective study of nature, as advocated by Grecian thinkers and adopted later by European minds, has given man a great deal of power over the laws of nature and made him successful in the attainment of pleasure. Without knowing the technique and value of concentration, these Occidental groups are often afraid even to think of it lest they lose their

---

[1] *Way of Perfection* (London: Thomas Baker, 1935), p. 91.

initiative and aggressiveness. Being, therefore, ignorant on this subject, they naturally fear what they do not understand.

There is also an erroneous idea that because Orientals generally practice concentration and meditation they have not attained worldly success. On the other hand, it is the prevailing impression that Occidental people, by their objective study of science and material progress, control physically not only Occidental life but Oriental life as well. It is not the intention to evaluate here the achievements of science and its pragmatic value in giving man real happiness and satisfaction. That is an entirely different question. Yet we are compelled to refute the unscientific conclusions of scientific thinkers and some of the religious leaders.

Our answer to the religious leaders is that the practice of meditation and concentration has been used not only by Oriental religious groups but also by Occidental religious groups such as the Christian mystics—St. Bernard, St. Ignatius, St. Teresa, and St. John of the Cross[2]—and many ancient and medieval Jewish mystics of Europe as well as Asia.[3] It is needless to say that Meister Eckhart, Thomas à Kempis, George Fox, John Wesley, and a number of other recent Christian leaders advocated certain forms of concentration and meditation.[4] It seems to us that it is impossible for a man to experience God without some form or practice of meditation. There may be divergence in the practices, yet one has to control the mind in order to have direct experience of the Ultimate Reality. One must remove the ego and selfishness to reach the goal of religion, whatever system one may choose. We know the Hindu view of the practices of

[2] Don Cuthbert Butler, *Western Mysticism* (London: Constable & Co., 1922).

[3] Gershom G. Scholem, *Major Trends in Jewish Mysticism* (Jerusalem: Schocken Publishing House, 1941).

[4] Rufus M. Jones, *Studies in Mystical Religion* (London: Macmillan & Co., 1923); and also Evelyn Underhill, *Mysticism* (7th ed.; London: Methuen & Co., Ltd., 1918).

meditation. In fact, everyone has to cleanse the mind to see God. We read in *Theologia Germanica*: "Furthermore, mark ye, that the one Being in whom God and man are united, standeth free of himself and of all things, and whatever is in him is there for God's sake and not for man's, or the creature's."[5] St. Thomas Aquinas says: "Therefore, in order to see God, there is needed some likeness of God on the part of the visual power, whereby the intellect is made capable of seeing God."[6]

Meditation does not make one passive or negative. On the contrary, it brings out the dynamic power of the mind. Only a man of meditation who has direct realization of God can successfully serve humanity. We have seen time and again that men and women start social service work with good intentions; yet in the course of actual performance they lose their high ideals and get mixed up with ambition, name, fame, and power. The history of religious and welfare organizations substantiates this observation. On the other hand, the people who conduct social service activities and at the same time practice concentration, meditation, and other devotional exercises can maintain the spirit of service and worship in and through their work. Some of the greatest men of meditation were the greatest servants of humanity, such as St. Francis of Assisi of Christian tradition and Swami Vivekananda of Hindu tradition. Buddha and his followers strongly advocated the practice of concentration and, at the same time, they were the people who flooded the ancient world with social service and unselfish work.

To the rationalistic thinkers we say that they should not come to any hasty conclusion about the effect of meditation without critical observation of the technique and its effect

[5] *Theologia Germanica,* trans. Susanna Winkworth (London: Macmillan & Co., 1874), p. 77.
[6] *Basic Writings of Saint Thomas Aquinas,* ed. by Anton C. Pegis (New York: Random House, 1944), I, p. 94.

on the human mind. Apart from its religious value, the practice of meditation has a tremendous influence in building up the total personality of man. We again mention that it really brings out the dynamic power of the mind with all its latent possibilities, as we said in the chapter on "Will and Personality." The conclusion is almost inevitable that without meditation the conflicts cannot be removed. Modern psychotherapy might help one temporarily, but it alone cannot give sufficient strength and stamina to the mind to ward off the evil influences of modern life.

It is true that the Occidental countries, with the help of scientific achievements, have done a great deal for the betterment of the everyday life of man. Yet in the West, because of the restlessness, unhappiness, and dissatisfaction of the mind, there are constant conflicts and frustrations resulting in extreme forms of mental disorders, nerve troubles, and functional ailments. This shows that the modern ways of life, based on scientific discoveries and their uses, have not solved the psychological problems of the West. On the other hand, the problems are becoming more and more frightening. So the West must find a way out of this dangerous situation.

It has been suggested by Jung that the Occidental people should develop a technique of their own for meditation. It is also implied by him that the minds of the Occidental people are different from those of the Orientals. On critical examination, we fully understand that the minds of Occidentals and Orientals are not different. There is no such thing as an Occidental mind and an Oriental mind. Psychological study will reveal that the actions and reactions of both groups are similar. A mother loves her child as intensely in the Orient as she does in the Occident. Hatred, jealousy, and envy are not the exclusive qualities of any one group. Intellectual achievements are also not to be found in one group alone. Above all, the spiritual experiences of man are the same in the Eastern countries as in the Western countries because of the similarity in mental attitudes and emotional expressions. The emotional devotees of Oriental countries, like Tulsidas and Mirabai, are similar to St. Anthony and St. Teresa. The intellectual type of spiritual realizations of Yajnavalkya, Sankara, and Swami Vivekananda is similar to that of St. Dionysius, St. Bernard, and Meister Eckhart. The differences in the type or form of spiritual achievements and realizations are due to the nature of the mind itself rather than to Oriental or Occidental habitation. For instance, the spiritual experiences of devotees approaching God through the emotions with love and devotion will be similar, but not the same as those of devotees approaching God through the intellect with reasoning and ratiocination. Spiritual decline has also occurred in the Eastern and Western civilizations, and great spiritual personalities have arisen in both parts of the world to revitalize the people. Buddha, Lao-Tze, Krishna, Sri Ramakrishna, and others again and again spiritualized the life of the Oriental countries and saved the people from utter materialism. Similarly, Christ, St. Francis, St. Bonaventure, and other great mystics saved the West from complete disintegration. It may be true that Western scientific and objective methods gave man the power to remove some of the onslaughts of nature and make him comfortable, but that does not prove at all that man's inner nature has been changed by scientific discoveries and achievements, or that the mind of a Westerner needs less meditation and religious exercises for the attainment of spiritual realizations than does the mind of an Oriental.

Apart from the religious values of the practice of concentration, there is a great deal of advantage in it so far as the psychological problems of modern man are concerned. Hindu psychologists classify mental states into five groups: (1) extreme restlessness, (2) partial restlessness, (3) dullness, (4) concentrated state, and (5) absolute concentration. All the modern psychologists fully realize that real satisfaction and happiness cannot be attained by a man unless he has overcome extreme restlessness. As a result, physicians and also psychotherapeutists greatly appreciate the need for mental stability in their patients; in fact, they prescribe definite methods for establishing a stable mind. Dr. Joseph Pratt of Boston, Dr. Carl G. Jung of Zurich, and many others operate mental clinics to give the patients mental training in relaxation and thought control. The doctors clearly relate how cases of physical ailments like toothache, "hysterical fever," psoriasis, and other diseases are being cured purely by psychological methods.[7]

There is a question in the minds of some of the experimental psychologists as to whether or not religious zeal and overemphasis on a religious ideal creates a fear complex and serious conflict. The real religious attitude cannot create any fear and conflict in the mind. On the contrary, a proper understanding of the values of religion removes the causes of fear and conflict. A sound philosophy helps us in overcoming the extreme restless and also the dull states of the mind. The practice of concentration creates interest in an aspect of God and so gradually helps to overcome restlessness.

Sometimes it is argued that this practice of meditation for a few minutes in the morning and evening would not stabilize a man's life, but experience proves that the steady practice of concentration for months and years does gradually stabilize the mind and creates a satisfaction which is the objective of psychotherapeutists. We cannot understand how the mere knowledge of conflicting emotions and of the causes of frustration can stabilize the mind. On the contrary, we find that people often get discouraged and disturbed over

[7] Carl G. Jung, *Psychology and Religion* (New Haven: Yale University Press, 1938), pp. 10-11.

the very causes of their conflicts, so it is imperative that their minds be trained to achieve at least partial concentration. This method also clarifies the higher values of life. It is observed that restlessness of the mind, due to conflict and frustration or any other such difficulty, creates serious physical disorders. We have observed that when a man practices concentration and meditation, he gradually overcomes extreme mental restlessness and spontaneously strengthens the nervous system, resulting in the proper functioning of the organs. Even from the therapeutic point of view, the practice of relaxation and concentration is of great importance, as illustrated by Dr. Joseph Pratt and his colleagues in the psychological clinic of the Boston Dispensary. They have proved that the practice of relaxation helps the patients in overcoming restlessness and eliminating functional disorders.

It is true that a higher philosophy of life is absolutely necessary for satisfactory living as it teaches us that all aspirations, hopes, and desires must be subordinated to the supreme goal of life, as previously explained. Effective understanding of a higher philosophy of life makes us see the necessity of regulating our inordinate affections and ambitions. On the other hand, the practice of relaxation and concentration is also absolutely essential. We may have philosophy; we may have theology; we may have religious principles; but they have to be applied in life individually through discipline, training, and exercises. History proves that philosophy does not become operative unless we apply it practically in our everyday life. The practice of concentration brings out the initiative of the mind so that we can make our philosophy dynamic. Every child knows that it is wrong to lie; every child knows that it is wrong to be angry; every man knows that it is vicious and harmful to be hateful or jealous; and every man knows that suspicion destroys him and his peace; yet no one can overcome these lower emotions if he has not the will power to apply the principles of religion and philosophy to his emotional reactions. The practice of concentration unifies the mind, strengthens the will, and enables one to apply these principles in his human behavior. Then his social contacts become harmonious, pleasant, and satisfactory.

We shall see the most important effect of concentration and meditation in the chapter on "Superconscious Experience." Suffice it to say that no person can have real spiritual knowledge or immediate awareness of God without being established in the methods of meditation. Mystics and spiritual aspirants may vary in their use of distinctive methods, yet they are all convinced of their utility.

CHAPTER VIII

Intuitive Insight

THERE is considerable confusion in the understanding of the intuitive faculty of man. Ordinary people often interpret the experiences of intuitive understanding as "sensing things." The term is often used loosely by the vast majority of the people. The real intuitive faculty is not expressed so easily and it requires considerable clarification in connection with the practice of meditation.

Intuitive insight is a state in which the mind becomes active in its totality. The practice of concentration harnesses all the mental powers and allows their forces to work in one direction. As a result, the whole mind becomes active and awakened when one achieves the absolute state of concentration. A man who has succeeded in attaining this absolute concentration in deep meditation has knowledge of the entire mind, and his mind becomes transparent and luminous. He does not need any objective study for the understanding of the subconscious states nor does he need any inferential knowledge of the hidden tendencies in the form of modern psychoanalysis. He detects immediately and directly the accumulated impressions of the mind that are embedded in the subconscious region, just as we see things in the showcase. Autognosis becomes the effect of direct perception. Moreover, there is an understanding of the total experience of the mind. A man does not then need to go to any other person for interpretation of his dreams or his behavior because he knows directly and immediately the constituent parts of his own total mind.

Apart from this, the most important achievement of the deep concentrated state and the highest intuitive insight is the experience of the Reality behind the objective world. When the rays of the sun are diffused, we do not get the full power of light or heat. On the other hand, when all the rays are converged, we get concentrated light and an intense form of heat. Similarly, when the mental forces are made restless, we do not understand the mind nor do we understand anything objectively. In extreme cases of restlessness, the mind becomes hopelessly inattentive and weak. But when the mental forces are converged upon one object, all the divergent elements are unified and the mind becomes extremely powerful. And that is the very reason that a man of deep meditation knows his total mind and, through its concentration, has the experience of Reality. As we observed in the lives of the great spiritual leaders belonging to different religions, the secret of their achievement lies in their one-pointedness of mind. They become so absorbed in God that they often forget even consciousness of the body.

When a man achieves this state of deep concentration, he can also direct his concentrated mind to other minds and understand immediately and directly their different states, just as one can see things objectively in the showcase of a department store. There is no mystery about understanding the minds of others. It becomes a fact of experience when a man achieves that concentrated state of mind. He does not have to interpret the behavior or dream of an individual in order to understand the cause of his actions nor does he need any inferential method to understand the subconscious tendencies of the person. He can know directly the impressions, however subtle they may be, in the mind of his friend or client. It is true that every man does not have that complete understanding and total use of the mind. The reason is not that it is impossible but rather that he has not developed absolute concentration of his mind, which is still being colored by objective experiences. Consequently, he is still restless. When a man achieves this absolute state of concentration and thereby his mind becomes colorless and transparent, then, and then alone, has he the knowledge of his own mind and also of the minds of others, if he so chooses.

Objective study and inferential knowledge of the contents of the unconscious mind are rather risky and apt to be unsound because the observer, in his interpretation of unknown subconscious impressions, cannot help coloring the interpretation by his own preconceived impressions and tendencies. Certain behavior may have different causes. A man may be restless because of his abnormal ambition, disappointment in friends, or because of his lack of self-expression, loss of money, failure in intellectual achievement, or for other reasons. It is but natural that an objective observer is likely to interpret the cause of restlessness and consequent nerve disorder through one or another of his own preconceived impressions. Unless an observer is a man of deep concentration, it is almost impossible for him to be unbiased. Consequently, he often becomes a failure in the interpretation of unconscious impressions and behavior complexes through the use of objective methods of dream interpretation and Freudian symbology.

The difference between intuitive insight and analytical objective knowledge should be discussed and evaluated here. Scientists objectively study the facts of experience through the methods of observation and experiment. In fact, they follow the method of "controlled experiment," as Professor Carlson and others mention, and find the laws and principles regarding the facts of experience. Most scientists seem to feel that this is the definite and positive method of knowledge; every fact is judged by this method. In general, Professor Carlson and other such materialistic and mechanistic scientists discard all other forms of knowledge. To them, intuitive knowledge of various kinds, including religious awareness, is superstition![1]

In our discussion and evaluation of the objective study of mind,[2] we found that it is difficult to know its inner workings by inferential objective study. Analysis of the emotional contents and subconscious urges is uncertain through objective interpretations of certain outer experiences. Of course, we do not minimize the importance of the analytical method and its place in certain areas of life. But it cannot be taken as the certitude of knowledge in all fields. Intuitive insight cannot be replaced by an analytical system in immediate and complete understanding of the mind and the Ultimate Reality. The inferential method based on objective study is extremely uncertain and vague. Professor Eddington, in his *Philosophy of Physical Science*, aptly comes to the conclusion that scientific knowledge of the analytical type is relative. Besides, it cannot give the knowledge of the Absolute which is beyond the categories of time, space, and causal relationships. It cannot give us knowledge of the "thing in itself" of philosopher Kant nor can it give us knowledge of the "Soul of the Universe" of Professor Stromberg. Philosophers like Kant, Herbert Spencer, and others are right in a sense when they say that the Ultimate Reality is unknown and unknowable, as it is beyond analytical empirical knowledge. But in another sense they are wrong, as the Ultimate Reality is more than unknown and unknowable; it is the very nature of the soul, of existence. However, it can be attained through development of intuitive apperception. Intuition plays a

---

[1] A. J. Carlson, "Science and the Supernatural," *Scientific Monthly*, LIX (August, 1944), 85-95.
[2] See Chapter IV, "The Subconscious Mind."

great part in religious experiences and higher phases of psychology.

Two questions naturally arise here. (1) Can we develop the intuitive faculty? (2) What is the test of its validity? Let us first consider the possibility of its development. It is true that some persons have "hunches" and intuitive understanding at times. A loving mother often instinctively knows when her child is in danger; she often does not require any external means of knowing it. Her inner feelings bespeak the condition of the child. We could give any number of illustrations, as many people have such experiences.

For instance, a mother told us recently that one night she was thinking incessantly of her son who was in the Pacific fighting zone, and she could not take her thoughts away from the boy. During the night she became very restless about him. She shivered violently and could not stop in spite of all the bedcovers she had over her. Suddenly, she felt a luminous presence in the room and heard a voice say: "Mother, everything is all right." The next morning she received a message from the government that her son's airplane had been shot down in the Pacific and the boy had been killed.

A prominent doctor reported to us a short while ago that a patient went to his office and told him that she had been extremely nervous about her husband that day. A message from Washington that night informed the doctor that the husband had had an airplane accident and had been killed.

Every loving soul understands the inner requirements of the beloved but it has no definite control over these experiences. Every time a child or husband is in danger, the mother or wife does not sense it. We may say that these experiences are "chance" and "coincidence"; they cannot be within the scope of scientific investigation. We admit that intuitive experiences are not usually under the control of the average man and woman, and our explanation is that their minds are not in a concentrated state in their ordinary everyday lives. Their minds are distracted and diffused, thinking successively of all sorts of things with no focus on any one thing for a period of time. Such minds do not become continuously and totally active. That is the reason they do not have intuitive insight as frequently as they would like to have it or should have it. However, under certain circumstances or conditions their minds do become totally active temporarily and they suddenly have intuitive knowledge. We have observed that the intuitive faculties of some people are developed without concentration. We cannot explain the cases scientifically; but, according to their belief in the theory of reincarnation, Hindu thinkers conclude that the intuitive faculties must have been developed in the previous life.

A person can systematically cultivate this faculty if he thoroughly practices concentration by learning to withdraw the mind from all sorts of activities and to focus it on one object regularly. He develops the power of directing the mind at his will as he chooses. Integration of will is one of the most important methods of cultivating intuition. Intuitive insight is fully developed in a man established in meditation, as we shall see in the next chapter.

Now let us consider the validity of its functioning. Although we know that there are genuine cases of intuitive insight, we fully realize that there are many persons who claim that they have it when they really have not; and they often judge others on this basis. The fact is that they often misjudge people and do injustice to them on the basis of this so-called insight and "sensing." Many of them create a great deal of trouble, confusion, and disturbance in life. It is unwise to depend on these hunches as facts unless we can test them carefully. Valid intuitive insight is present in a person who is thoroughly integrated and whose will is unified and made entirely active by being established in higher principles of ethics and practice of deep concentration and meditation. When we observe the life of the individual carefully, then we can test the insight. In fact, we can safely conclude that the claim of intuitive insight is trustworthy and dependable only when the mind is unified and made totally active through training and discipline. Otherwise, an occasional release of insight may be true at times yet it cannot be trusted or regarded as valid unless it is verified.

CHAPTER IX

Extrasensory Experiences

MOST ordinary people and many scientists assume that conscious and sensuous experiences are the only realities in the world. However, there are some experiences in human life which are not connected with immediate sense perception. These are generally named in various ways. Some of them are called telepathy, extrasensory perception, miracles, supernatural phenomena, and mystic or religious experiences. They were not studied by scientific minds until Professor William James of Harvard University collected, compiled, and classified some of them as religious experiences. Most of the psychologists ridiculed these extraordinary experiences studied by Professor James and often called them pathological states. We are happy that he collected these facts for general observation and study in a thoroughgoing and scientific way. He did not ridicule them nor show any preconceived notion or prejudice against them. Rather he submitted them for fair and dispassionate study and investigation.

There are critics of these extraordinary happenings among religious groups as well as outside them. It is admitted that these unusual experiences of man cannot be observed objectively as they are not generally repeated for controlled observation at the convenience of the investigators. Yet it is the height of folly to ridicule or condemn them without thorough scientific investigation. There are a few advanced societies, like the Society for Psychical Research, that are trying to investigate some of these phenomena. They have studied such experiences and have collected some undeniable facts which fall within the scope of the science of psychology.

We do not mean to say that all the claims of such extraordinary and extrasensory experiences are valid. There have been many unjustifiable statements which were not verified and supported by facts. So we cannot blame anyone for being skeptical and critical about them. We ourselves are also critical and discourage mystery mongering. Such indulgence demoralizes and confuses the minds of the people, and it often makes them gullible and superstitious. As a rule we do not condemn them, as Professor Carlson would have us do, but we advocate a critical attitude and openness of mind so that we can actually find the truth about them. The attitude should be scientific in all the investigations. Psychology as a science should also have the true spirit of observation and investigation as expressed by Professor James and Professor Müller-Freienfels, even though these experiences cannot be repeated for the purpose of controlled observation. For that matter, there are many facts in our mental life which cannot always be objectified, as, for instance, the actual contents of emotional reactions.

Professor Rhine in his book, *New Frontiers of the Mind*, describes some of these extrasensory experiences of man and has tried to develop a technique for understanding them. He and some of his colleagues have come to the conclusion that the mind has certain powers for getting knowledge other than through the usual nerve reactions. McDougall seems also to be sympathetic to this system of investigation. It is true that ordinary perceptions are gathered through the nervous system, but extraordinary experiences are achieved without direct contact of the sense organs and nervous system. Yet they have exact and immediate value so far as the experience is concerned, the same value as if they had been acquired through the senses. They are not imaginative and poetic flights but are of practical value, as they furnish new knowledge of certain facts. These experiences fall within the range of immediate knowledge as opposed to inferential knowledge. Although they may or may not have a connection with religious experiences, many religious persons who have higher mystic realizations also have these extrasensory perceptions.

Let us examine a few instances in which such perceptions have actually taken place. The daughter of a friend of ours, who is a great medical man and authority in this section of the country, had a peculiar or extraordinary experience when she was about thirteen years old. She called her mother one night after she had gone to bed and reported that she smelled something burning in the house. The mother made light of the statement and asked the little girl to go back to bed and rest. After a few minutes the child called again and insisted that she could smell the burning of flesh. The mother at once got out of bed and went around the house but found no trace of fire; so she advised the daughter to go to sleep and told her that perhaps she had been dreaming. In a short while the girl came out of her room and insisted that she detected a very strong odor of something burning, but the mother could do nothing about it. Early the next morning they received a telephone call from a city about a hundred miles away, bringing the news that during the previous night one of the nearest relatives of the mother had been burned alive by a fire which destroyed the home. This very experience and other such experiences definitely suggest that a human being can have direct perception of something that is happening at a distant place without direct contact through the senses or the nervous system.

A friend was sitting with us in our living room and we were both reading. She suddenly declared: "There will be a death in this house," and burst into tears. I told her that I had no indication that I would die in the near future nor had I any feeling that her daughter or any of my friends or anyone else would die suddenly. So I tried to console her. About three days later in the course of our service a man, who had just played some music, suddenly had a heart attack and died within a few minutes. This experience of my friend in foreseeing the death is an undeniable fact which we witnessed and which was verified by all who attended the service. This same friend, while staying in India, on one occasion suddenly told me that there would be a death. She had an immediate experience of that future happening. After a day or two we received a cable from America that one of our Swamis, who was a very dear friend of mine, had passed on. This friend had the same type of experience on another occasion regarding a death which took place within a short time.

We know of many cases in India in which men and women know future events, like death or disease, directly and immediately without coming in direct contact with the occurrence through the nervous system or senses. There are people in all parts of the world who are unusually constituted and understand future happenings immediately and directly even before the occurrence of the incidents. We know some other cases intimately in America, India, and other places, the validity of which cannot be denied, as they were verified by actual events.

Many of us know that thoughts can be transferred to a distant place. Some persons are emotionally attuned in such a way that they can transfer their thoughts and emotions to one another without speaking or being directly in touch with each other. An American friend of ours often used to tell us that he and his mother were so close they did not have to talk or express their thoughts and emotions; each would know the other's thoughts and feelings directly and would act accordingly. Again, we often hear of friends or parents and children who became aware of sickness, one of the other, through mental telepathy, even though they may have been in different places or in separate countries.

In the chapters on "Will and Personality" and "Intuitive Insight" we described some of the extraordinary powers by which a man can control the ordinary laws of nature, like the burning quality of fire; and we know cases of suspension of animation. We also know of cases of emanation of light and other such powers.[1] There is no need to illustrate these further, although many such events which were verified could be mentioned. Generally these are regarded by religious groups as miracles or divine visitations. For instance, the extraordinary happenings in the life of Jesus, the Christ, are regarded in Western countries as divine power displayed through Him. Western devotees often understand these manifestations as miracles in some of their Christian or Jewish mystics.

Hindu psychologists, like Patanjali and others, discovered laws of the mind which explain such extraordinary occurrences. Extrasensory perceptions or occult powers are not miracles nor are they accidental; they are governed and controlled by subtle mental laws. Western psychology by ridiculing and ignoring these facts is losing an opportunity of studying some interesting mental phenomena. Indian psychology, on the other hand, took account of these extraordinary powers and developed methods by which they can be experienced and manifested by everyone. It seems to us that Western psychology is narrow and partial in ignoring and condemning these phenomena without thorough scientific

---

[1] Swami Saradananda, *Sri Sri Ramakrishna Lilaprasanga*, II.

investigation. We admit that there are some difficulties in scientific investigation, as the methods of development of these extraordinary powers are quite different from the methods that are adopted by the physical sciences. The methods that are used both to manifest and verify such powers are purely subjective and internal. Patanjali gives an elaborate description of these phenomena and also the ways in which one can develop them through prescribed methods of concentration on certain objects. He also explains that some persons are born with these tendencies and others can cultivate them by systematic practice.[2]

It is necessary now to say a word regarding the criticism of these extraordinary powers. We go to a chemist with chemical problems, and he has to apply certain methods which are suitable to the investigation of chemical facts. On the other hand, a biologist will take up quite a different method for his investigation, while an astronomer will apply his telescope and other apparatus for the study of astronomical data. We cannot apply astronomical apparatus to biology or physics. Similarly, psychological facts can be investigated only by psychological methods. So Patanjali prescribes such methods with which to develop mental power. *If anyone wants to investigate these extraordinary powers of extrasensory experiences, he must come to the same state of development as the persons who manifest them. Without having the required mental power it would be impossible for a person to observe and evaluate properly such subtle displays of extrasensory perceptions and occult powers.* It seems to us the height of folly on the part of scientists to ridicule these experiences without thorough investigation. We certainly advocate that the experimenter be thoroughly trained as well as the person studied, so that we can have a proper and correct evaluation, just as the jeweler, and not

[2] *Yoga Aphorisms of Patanjali*, chap. III.

the grocer, can properly evaluate a jewel. We, too, want to be critical in our observation.

There are abnormal persons who talk of visions and extraordinary experiences, but those claimed experiences are mere figments of their minds. They have delusions and hallucinations about certain events and also about themselves. People who have delusions and hallucinations show symptoms of mental disintegration. Their emotions are not controlled, their nerves are shattered, and they are much inferior to an average person. A little critical study will reveal that such persons are abnormal and belong to the department of psychopathy. Many psychopathic cases have such extraordinary illusions and hypnotic spells that they seem to live in a dreamland. It is quite evident that they do not have normal integration of mind, and their behavior is vitiated by their fancies and imaginary perceptions. *The real criterion is the effect on the character of the person.* If we observe that the claimed experiences have weakened the personality and demoralized the individual, then these experiences are mere figments of the imagination.

This does not mean that all extrasensory perceptions are within the realm of hallucination, however. We can easily differentiate between hallucinations and actual extrasensory perceptions by a critical test of the validity of their effects and by a study of the character of the person involved. The same scientific test will prove when extrasensory perceptions are valid and when they are only figments of an unstable mind. In the case of hallucinations no new information is added to the fund of knowledge. A person who has them is often confused, while in extrasensory perception new knowledge of a fact or event is gained.

Patanjali, in his description of the various extrasensory powers and methods of attaining them, states definitely that they are great obstacles to higher spiritual experiences and mystic realizations. As we have already related, Buddha, Sri Ramakrishna, and others strongly discouraged the use of occult powers. They also said that if anyone wants to have higher spiritual realizations he must discourage preoccupation with extraordinary phenomena, although these may occur simultaneously with spiritual practices. In fact, we know intimately that in the course of some intense spiritual practices one sometimes unconsciously and unintentionally develops these powers. A real teacher of spiritual life always advises his disciple to stop their manifestation; otherwise, the mind of the disciple would be lowered to the level of these powers instead of being lifted to the divine plane.[3]

[3] *Yoga Aphorisms of Patanjali* III:51.

CHAPTER X

The Superconscious State

SPIRITUAL experiences or superconscious visions, as well as meditation, are criticized and questioned by some of the religious groups and scientific thinkers. In the first place, the criticism is that mystic realizations make one other-worldly and cause him to be what they call an "introvert;" that is to say, these experiences make one forget his fellow beings and become self-centered. They seem to think that the most important fact of religious life is to do good to others. They advocate what some of them term the "social gospel," which is based on the maxim "Love thy neighbor." They do not wholly refute the utility of prayers but they advocate that people should not give much time to them. A man serves God when he does good to other fellow beings, establishes social justice and economic stability for all, and removes the evils from society. That is, indeed, a noble sentiment, but these religious groups and scientific thinkers miss the real objective of religious life. Jesus gave the first commandment: "And thou shalt love the Lord thy God with all thy heart, and with all thy soul, and with all thy mind, and with all thy strength." And His second commandment was: "Thou shalt love thy neighbor as thyself."[1]

Let us not forget that the aim and goal of religion is to know and experience God or the Ultimate Reality. If any-

[1] Mark 12:30 and 31, and Matt. 22:37 and 39.

one or any group ignores the first commandment of Jesus, he is bound to miss the primary objective of religion. The religious history of the world proves to us that whenever the persons or groups, especially religious groups, forget the primary objective of life, they invariably become social and political in character. In course of time, the original understanding of even the second commandment changes. The enthusiasm for social welfare gradually becomes lukewarm and the fervor dies. Contemporary history emphatically proves it.

The humanists of modern Europe and America deny completely the meaning of the first commandment and ignore the utility of prayer, not to speak of meditation. Religious experiences and superconscious visions are wholly unknown and unthought of by them. It is sufficient to say that they completely forget the main problem of religious life. It should be mentioned that, although both scientific and religious humanists forget that religion must lead one to the knowledge of the Ultimate Reality or God, they are good people and strongly advocate ethical living and social welfare. However, we make bold to say that ethics is not the goal of religion, although one cannot grow spiritually unless one is thoroughly established in the highest ethical principles, as explained in the chapter on "Meditation." Hindu psychologists and religious leaders are emphatic on this point; they say that a person cannot be fit to meditate unless he lives an ethical life, nay, unless he overcomes the causes of mental agitation. The causes of mental disturbances are the lower tendencies of man—hatred, envy, jealousy, greed, lust, love of power, egotism, and other such negative qualities. We advise every critic of Hindu philosophy and religion to note that a man is not considered fit to discuss higher spiritual questions and to inquire into the nature of God or Brahman unless he is established in *shama* and *dama*, internal and external purification.[2]

And he who is devoid of proper understanding, thoughtless and always impure, never attains that goal, and gets into the round of births and deaths.

But he who is intelligent, ever pure and with the mind controlled, reaches that goal whence none is born again.[3]

Ethical living is absolutely necessary for religious experiences and superconscious vision. We will also see that as a man has these experiences he grows immensely in higher ethical principles; he cannot have valid superconscious experiences and be unethical or nonethical. Moreover, these experiences are far higher than just ethical living. In fact, a man of superconscious realization is the veritable embodiment of ethics.

True social service, philanthropic work, and love of neighbor are practiced and taught by the people who are well established in these higher experiences and love of God. So the refutations of some religious groups and scientific thinkers are far from the truth. The real mystic who has spiritual realizations or superconscious experiences becomes extremely interested in his fellow beings as he finds the expression of God in them. A mystic feels the presence of God everywhere and so he takes a loving interest not only in human beings but also in other beings. St. Francis of Assisi, after having his mystic realizations, saw first the presence of God in every object; and secondly, he could feel universal brotherhood everywhere. He could even change ferocious animals into gentle creatures by his loving expressions. Similarly, in India there are persons who have changed the lives of human beings and other beings by their very loving expressions which came out of the depth of their mystic realizations. Swami

---

[2] This is explained in *Katha Upanishad* and other Upanishads; *Vedanta Sutra; Vivekachudamani* by Sri Sankaracharya; and *Yoga Aphorisms.*

[3] *Katha Upanishad* 3:7 and 8.

Vivekananda, Swami Brahmananda, and others became the true awakeners of Indian culture and the true servants of humanity because of their intense spiritual realizations that brought out their love for humanity. When you study the lives of Christian, Hindu, Buddhist, and Mohammedan mystics, and other religious personalities, you will find that the secret of their loving service lies in the depth of their mystic superconscious experiences.

Another point of criticism is that these religious experiences only occur abnormally and pathologically. This criticism has been made since time immemorial. All of the great spiritual personalities were at some time or other regarded as pathological. It is true that such experiences are rare. Ordinary people have no conception of them. Besides, they are far beyond the scope of the experiences which were discussed in the previous chapter. These so-called extrasensory perceptions, including telepathy and occult and psychic powers, are of a lower type and should not be confused with superconscious visions and realizations. These extraordinary powers do not give us the knowledge of the Reality or God and, as such, they have practically no value in religious research. In fact, as we have explained in the previous chapter, they often become obstacles. They do, however, give some information on certain subtle realms of consciousness, even without having any connection with experiences of the Ultimate Reality; while, on the other hand, superconscious visions lead direct to the realization of the Real or God. The average man cannot understand the superconscious. According to the *Gita*: "That which is night to all beings, in that the Self-controlled man wakes. That in which all beings wake, is night to the Self-seeing Muni" (man of realization).[4] Therefore, God-vision is not abnormal nor is it created by an insane mentality. Swami Saradananda gives us a critical evaluation

[4] *Srimad-Bhagavad-Gita* II:6a.

of these experiences, showing that those who have had them are transformed personalities.[5] He declares that the ordinary man cannot experience them without regular training and steady spiritual practices. These realizations make one pure and gradually give one infinite joy.

So we find that they are not abnormal, but rather they are supernormal. In abnormal cases we find that a man's mind is disintegrated; his emotions have no harmony; his intellect and emotions do not co-ordinate; and his actions are incongruous and inconsistent. In every way abnormal persons are far inferior to average persons. On the contrary, one who has experienced superconscious realization attains complete integration of mind; his emotions are fully controlled; his intellect, emotions, and will are co-ordinated. In fact, a man cannot have higher superconscious experiences unless his mind is wholly controlled and disciplined. As Swami Brahmananda says:

This mind cannot know Him. He is beyond this mortal mind and far beyond the human intellect. This apparent universe which you see is within the domain of the mind. The mind is its author, the mind has conjured it up. It cannot go beyond its own domain.

Behind the mind of which we are aware is a subtle, spiritual mind, existing in seed-form. Through contemplation, prayer, and *japam* [repetition of the name of God], this mind develops and with its unfoldment a new vision opens. The aspirant realizes many spiritual truths. However, this is not the final experience. This subtle mind also cannot reach God, the Supreme Atman. But it leads you nearer to Him. At this stage the world loses all its charm for the aspirant. He remains absorbed in the consciousness of God.

Next comes samadhi. The experience of samadhi is indescribable—beyond *is* and *is not*. In this blessed experience there is

[5] Swami Saradananda, *Sri Sri Ramakrishna Lilaprasanga*, II, 44.

neither happiness nor misery, neither light nor darkness. All is Infinite Being—inexpressible.[6]

Patanjali emphasizes the practice of controlling the mental states in his discussion of *Raja Yoga*. According to him, *yoga* (state of union or *samadhi*) is attained by perfect mental control.[7] Swami Vivekananda was never tired of showing the necessity of mental control, meaning ultimate transformation rather than repression. He says:

Most of us make our minds like spoiled children, allowing them to do whatever they want. Therefore it is necessary that *Kriya-yoga* [spiritual exercises] should be constantly practiced, in order to gain control of the mind, and bring it into subjection. The obstructions to *Yoga* [superconscious realization] arise from lack of control, and cause us pain. They can only be removed by denying the mind, and holding it in check, through the means of *Kriya-yoga*.[8]

The Christian mystics and others also emphatically insist on the necessity of mental training. According to St. Thomas Aquinas:

This light is required to see the divine essence, not as a likeness in which God is seen, but as a perfection of the intellect, strengthening it to see God. Therefore it may be said that this light is not a medium *in which* God is seen, but one *by which* He is seen; and such a medium does not take away the immediate vision of God.[9]

St. Teresa says:

Since you do not continue in your work according to your own personal plans, you need not fear lest your labor be in vain. Observe what I say, that we are all to strive for Him, because we

[6] *The Eternal Companion*, p. 100.
[7] *Yoga Aphorisms of Patanjali* I:2 and II:2.
[8] *Works*, I, 237.
[9] *St. Thomas Aquinas*, I, 99.

are not here for any other purpose. Strive, not for one or two years only, not even for ten, lest it should appear that we are quitting like cowards.[10]

Brother Lawrence also speaks of mental discipline:

I cannot imagine how religious persons can live satisfied without the practice of *the presence of* God.

. . . .

Let it be *your* business to keep the mind in the presence of the Lord. If it sometimes wander and withdraw itself from Him, do not much disquiet yourself for that: trouble and disquiet serve rather to distract the mind than to recollect it; the will must bring it back in tranquillity.[11]

It is meaningless to say that these are Oriental ideas alone. They are common ideas of all deeply spiritual persons who have superconscious realization. This shows that criticism against superconscious experiences is not based on facts and is, consequently, unscientific.

Another objection has been made that these so-called superconscious experiences are epileptic fits and, consequently, expressions of abnormalities of mind and body. Our answer is that in an epileptic fit or swoon a man loses his consciousness, and after the fit his whole nervous system and mind are affected and made weaker. It can be said definitely that he does not gain anything in the seizure and he acquires no new knowledge. The effect is often the same as from narcotics. On the other hand, a man enters into the superconscious state as an ordinary person and comes out of it a better man. His entire personality is transformed; his emotions are wholly controlled; he is master of himself; his will is extremely dynamic; he can achieve what he wills to do;

---

[10] Translated by Professor Edgar S. Brightman from *Camino de Perfección* [*The Way of Perfection*] (1881), Cop. XVIII, parts of 1 and 2, p. 57.

[11] Brother Lawrence, *The Practice of the Presence of God* (New York: Fleming H. Revell Co., 1895), pp. 32 and 35.

and he gains knowledge which he never previously had. Swami Vivekananda makes it clear in *Raja Yoga* that sleep, epileptic seizure, and any such state is beneath the conscious plane. On the other hand, superconsciousness is far above it. He says:

What makes the difference? From one state a man comes out the very same man that he went in, and from another state the man comes out enlightened, a sage, a prophet, a saint, his whole character changed, his life changed, illumined. These are the two effects. Now the effects being different, the causes must be different. As this illumination with which a man comes back from *Samadhi* is much higher than can be got from unconsciousness, or much higher than can be got by reasoning in a conscious state, it must therefore be super-consciousness, and *Samadhi* is called the super-conscious state.[12]

It is interesting to note what St. Teresa of Avila had to say in this connection. She emphatically answers the critics of all ages. She says:

If a vision were a mere product of one's own mind . . . it would be like the experience of a person who tried to put himself to sleep yet stays awake, because sleep has not come. He yearns for it, . . . he gets drowsy, he tries his best, and occasionally he seems to have accomplished something. But if it is not true sleep, it will not refresh him nor give strength to his head. In fact, it may leave him dizzier. It is the same way, to some extent, in the case of the soul. [If the vision were a product of the mind's effort], the soul would remain confused, not sustained and strengthened, but tired and disgusted. But in the real vision, it is impossible to exaggerate the riches of the soul and the health and comfort of the body which remain after the experience. . . . I resorted to this and other reasoning, when they told me that it was a devil [that gave me my visions], and that they were mere fancies— however often I experienced them, and I cited illustrative in-

[12] *Works*, I, 181.

G*

stances. . . . I said to them once, that if those who talked thus to me were to tell me that a person who had just finished talking to me, and whom I knew well, was not that person, but that I was indulging in fancies (as they knew), then I should doubtless believe those people rather than what I had seen. But if that person had left some jewels with me, and if, when I had had no jewels before, these remained in my hands as pledges of great love; if I, who was poor, beheld that I was rich—then I could not believe those who discredited my experience, even if I wanted to. I could show these jewels; everyone who knew me would see clearly that my soul was different. My father-confessor said so. The difference was very great in all things. It was no dissimulation, but everyone could see it clearly. . . . I myself saw clearly that I had suddenly become a different person through these visions.[13]

The superconscious experiences not only change the intellectual side of the mind by giving it a new fund of knowledge of the reality behind the phenomenal world, but they also change the quality of the emotional life of a person. A mind that has had superconscious experience needs no inference or logic to understand the existence of God. It immediately experiences and senses that Reality and has dynamic conviction of the existence of God and soul. The intellect is fully illumined, and the emotions are integrated and satisfied. There is great refinement and exaltation of the contents of the emotional side of the mind of a man of such realizations. His happiness knows no bounds, for he has reached the culmination of consciousness—the mine of bliss. His whole inner life is extremely peaceful, so much so that everyone can feel the radiance of peace and bliss.[14]

[13] Translated by Professor Edgar S. Brightman from *La Vida de La Santa Madre Terasa de Jesus*, Cop. 28, parts of 10 and 11, in D. Vecinti de Fuenti, *Abras de Santa Terasa de Jesus* (1881), Vol. I. pp. 165-66.

[14] *The Gospel of Sri Ramakrishna*, trans. Swami Nikhilananda (New York: Ramakrishna-Vivekananda Center, 1942); and *Sayings of Sri Ramakrishna* (2nd ed.; Mylapore, Madras).

It is often argued that religion only gives us the higher values of life by teaching us moral principles. However, it stabilizes society by establishing moral values of equality and brotherhood which promise harmonious living. Even objective scientific thinkers would accept this value of religion from the pragmatic and utilitarian point of view. It is indeed true that religion furnishes higher values of life. But this is not its primary contribution. Superconscious realizations reveal new experiences hitherto unknown to people. They give direct and immediate knowledge of the Reality or God. Truth is attained in its integral unity. One understands the basic unity of existence. A survey of the superconscious realizations of Sri Ramakrishna will prove to us that a flood of knowledge comes to a man of religious experiences.[15] It will also prove that these experiences are verifiable by following the methods of mental discipline and training. In fact, these superconscious experiences can be attained by anyone provided he goes through the required exercises.[16]

Just as the scientists make no claim that the possibility for verification of scientific truth is the exclusive property of a particular race or country, so also there is no exclusive right to the supreme knowledge of God. Any man belonging to any religion, race, or country can attain the same types of superconscious experiences. As we shall see in the next chapter, he may follow different methods according to the individual characteristics of his mind—whether they are devotional, meditative, intellectual, or active—and not because he belongs to a specific place or group.

It is also often said that these experiences may not be actual pathological conditions; yet they may be projections of one's thoughts, products of creative imagination, or instances

[15] *Life of Sri Ramakrishna* (3rd ed.; Mayavati, Almora, Himalayas: Advaita Ashrama, 1929).
[16] *Sayings of Sri Ramakrishna*, chap. XIX.

of self-hypnosis and autosuggestion. Some say that many children with creative imagination often talk with imaginary persons and have great fun with them as a result of such states of mind. These critics seem to think that superconscious experiences are similar to such childish imagination, and they are more tolerant than others, feeling pity rather than antagonism toward those who claim to have them. In their opinion such persons are laboring under delusion and are living in an imaginative world or in hallucination. Therefore, they try to remove the so-called "spell" of imagination or hallucination by giving them right understanding. But critical evaluation of superconscious experiences convinces us that they can be construed neither as pathological states nor as products of imagination, hallucination, or autosuggestion. If such were the case, the effects would not be elevating, as already described. Autosuggestion can bring a person to a state of oblivion and stupor where he lives in a dream world. On the contrary, superconscious experience gives definite new knowledge and transforms the personality, which could not be accomplished by self-hypnosis and creative imagination. However powerful imagination or suggestion may be, it cannot give more than the mind contains nor can it change the personality by integrating the emotions. Superconscious realization expands our consciousness and illumines us, giving real knowledge of the Absolute or God. As described in *Theologia Germanica*:

Moreover there are yet other ways to the lovely life of Christ, besides those we have spoken of: to wit, that God and man should be wholly united, so that it can be said of a truth, that God and man are one. This cometh to pass on this wise. Where the Truth always reigneth, so that true perfect God and true perfect man are at one. . . .[17]

[17] *Theologia Germanica*, pp. 75-76.

We feel that the experiences achieved by Sri Ramakrishna, Christ, Buddha, Krishna, and lesser personalities are really the basis of social values. A man ought to be just and loving because of the experience of unity of life and existence. Equality, brotherhood, and such other principles are really based on these facts of knowledge. In fact, religious experiences of this type are the true fundamentals of social service. The man who has these realizations is really capable of serving his fellow beings because he experiences the unity of life and existence. This is the background of "love thy neighbor." The lofty ethical ideas, that we appreciate and advocate, are the outcome of the higher realizations of men and women belonging to different religions.

So we see that superconscious experiences do not merely give us higher values of life but they also give us new funds of knowledge which we previously did not have. This knowledge is not only unique and new, it is also universal and verifiable by anyone who desires to go through the required training. Besides, this unique knowledge really furnishes the background and *raison d'être* of the higher values of life in the form of love of neighbors, brotherhood, and equality. Liberty, equality, and fraternity are taught by men of such experiences. We make bold to say that they cannot be established in human society unless they are inspired, strengthened, and guided by men of such realization. Contemporary history proves to us that love is not manifest in them, and mere talk of religion and God does not help us to achieve them. Only those whose character is based on superconscious experience can inspire a society to establish universal brotherhood and show what real love is. They do not talk of love but they manifest it in a dynamic form in and through their lives and actions, as we have already mentioned. They are the God-intoxicated lovers of God and man.

Samadhi or superconscious experiences may be classified

in different groups as described by Patanjali[18] and other great authorities like Sri Ramakrishna.[19] The life and experiences of this great personality reveal many extremely interesting facts of spiritual realization. There are many experiences which cannot be regarded as *samadhi* proper, yet they are "the milestones on the way to progress," as Swami Vivekananda calls them. These experiences are visions of divine forms or personal aspects of God, and they are of various types according to the mental constitution of the individual.[20] There are innumerable such experiences, and they convince a seeker of truth that he is on the right path. It should be noted here that all devotees do not have the same experiences and visions. In fact, some may not have any of them. Yet they may be progressing toward superconscious realization as they are becoming purer, more unselfish, and more loving. They invariably manifest spiritual qualities whether or not they have these visions.

However, there are persons who conclude that if anyone does not have these extraordinary experiences he is not evolving spiritually. This view is often expressed by sincere persons. Many devotees get discouraged on the path of spiritual life if they have no visions. We are told that, at times, some of the disciples expressed discouragement to Sri Ramakrishna. Once one of them noticed that his brother disciples and other devotees were having different types of spiritual experiences and even *samadhi*, but he had none. He approached Sri Ramakrishna, who encouraged him, saying that such experiences are not the criteria of spiritual growth. The real test is in the manifestation of love, devotion, conviction, and mental strength and purity. Of course, later on this disciple, too, had *samadhi*.

[18] *Yoga Aphorisms of Patanjali*, chap. I.
[19] *Gospel of Sri Ramakrishna* (5th ed.; Mylapore, Madras: Sri Ramakrishna Math, 1930), I, 87-123.
[20] Swami Saradananda, *Sri Sri Ramakrishna Lilaprasanga*, II, chap. 2.

We are fully aware that there is considerable criticism of extraordinary experiences by scientific minds. We cannot blame them, as there are so many questionable cases and stories which make one skeptical. However, as we previously stated, one should not ignore all the experiences just because of the false cases. Our answer to critics is that the valid experiences change the character of a person. He gradually manifests higher ethical and spiritual qualities. The effect is the best test and real proof of their validity. Moreover, they can be verified by every individual if he trains himself properly, as we shall understand in the following chapters.

When the devotees reach higher levels of spiritual growth, they attain the different stages of *samadhi* or superconscious states. There are many gradations even in the various types of *samadhi*. *Savikalpa samadhi* gives the experience of the personal aspect of God. In this a man has the direct and immediate knowledge of the personal aspect of God while he remains separate from the object of worship or love. There is duality in the experience. Various expressions of the body and mind occur at the time of absorption in the ideal; a man loses all consciousness of the physical world yet he is fully aware of the enjoyment which he receives from the realization. Outwardly it may appear that he is in something similar to a fit, or he is unconscious; yet he is fully conscious of the object that he is experiencing. His whole mind is completely withdrawn from the objective world and is focused on the object of realization. It is true that he is unconscious of the objective world; nevertheless, he is fully aware of the subtle inner world. In this state a devotee remains well established in one of the loving relationships with the personal aspect of God (*Ishta*). A devotee takes God as mother, father, child, friend, or beloved and thereby becomes absorbed in Him. In this form of *samadhi*, love reaches its culmination; and as such, it makes the devotee the veritable embodiment of love.

It often happens that a devotee who attains *savikalpa samadhi* through an intense form of love gradually attains other forms of *samadhi*.

In the superconscious state of *nirvikalpa samadhi* the individual transcends the limitation of personality and immediately and directly experiences the Absolute in its integral unity. His soul is completely identified with the Absolute. The knower, known, and knowledge become one (*Triputi Veda*). One of the *Upanishads* says: "As a result of meditation, the enjoyer, the enjoyed, and the power which brings about enjoyment—all are declared to be the three aspects of Brahman."[21] In other words, all differences and their relations merge into *one*. As Jesus said: "I and my Father are one." Hindu teachers say: "I am Brahman." These statements are from the depth of the realization of oneness with the Absolute. In that state a man also remains fully unconscious of the objective world, even of his own body, yet inwardly he is one with Consciousness Itself. His whole inner life is changed, and he has identified himself with the whole of existence. All limitations of time, space, and causation and the categories of objective knowledge are completely negated and annulled. What remains then is pure existence, pure knowledge, and pure bliss. All the contents of the empirical self are completely swept away and what remains is the pure Self (*Atma*). Swami Brahmananda briefly gives a clear idea:

Samadhi is generally classified as of two kinds. In *savikalpa*, the first sort of *samadhi*, there is the mystic vision of a spiritual form of God, while the consciousness of individuality still remains. In *nirvikalpa*, the other type of *samadhi*, a man loses his individuality and goes beyond the vision of the form of God. The whole universe then disappears. There is yet another kind called *Ananda* (blissful) *samadhi*. If an ordinary man reaches

[21] *Svetasvatara Upanishad* 1:12.

this experience, his body and brain cannot bear the supreme ecstatic joy. He does not live more than twenty-one days.[22]

The outer expression of these different types of superconscious experiences varies in different individuals. There are some physical changes and expressions which are regarded as manifestations of higher spiritual emotions in the body.[23] These are the physical indications of higher inner growth. One, however, must not confuse these with the goal of life. They are only the signs of progress. The greater the man, the greater his control of outer physical symptoms. It is interesting to note that the great Christian mystic, St. Teresa of Avila, expresses a similar idea. She says:

> The best sign that anyone has made progress is that she thinks herself the last of all and proves it by her behavior, and that she aims at the well being and good of others in all she does. This is the truest test.[24]

Bhava and various types of *samadhi* vary greatly in different individuals, and these persons are classified accordingly. They are called *Jivan Muktas* (liberated souls) of various types according to the depth of their experiences.[25] Their power of love also differs according to the gradation of their realizations. Again, it is observed that they vary in their power to change the lives of others. Some can transform a number of persons while others change a whole society; and there are some who actually usher in a new civilization and change the thought current of the world by their own life and character. Their own transformed personality is so dynamic that they become the center of a new civilization. Sri Krishna, Buddha, Christ, Sri Ramakrishna, and others

[22] *The Eternal Companion*, p. 107.
[23] These are the eightfold physical expressions of inner *bhavas* (spiritual emotions).
[24] *Way of Perfection*, p. 107.
[25] *Gospel of Sri Ramakrishna*, I, 87-123.

belong to this group. They are the builders of civilization. The power they exert lies in complete union with the Absolute. The ordinary devotees cannot remain in those extraordinary states of superconsciousness for a long time, as we understand from the *Gospel of Sri Ramakrishna* and the teachings of Swami Brahmananda which we have quoted. But the Incarnations remain absorbed in blissful *samadhi* from which they emerge time and again to help humanity. One who has even a glimpse of *bhava* or a lower form of spiritual experience is amazed to realize such a blissful state. A man of experience can alone appreciate this with joyous wonderment. We again say that modern science is baffled in the understanding of these experiences. But we request the scientist to go through the required training and verify them himself!

Professor Jung in his book, *Integration of the Personality*, states that this superconscious experience is a deep unconscious state.

There are dreams and visions of such an informative kind that the people who have them refuse to believe that they are derived from an unconscious psyche. They prefer to suppose that they issue from a sort of superconscious. Such people usually distinguish between a quasi-physiological or instinctive, unconscious and a psychic sphere or logos, "above" consciousness which they style the superconsciousness. As a matter of fact, the psyche called the superior or the universal in Hindu philosophy, corresponds to what the West calls the unconscious.[26]

He further says:

The yogis wind up with *Samadhi* an ecstatic condition that seems to be equivalent to an unconscious state. . . . A universal consciousness is logically identical with the unconscious . . . but the contents of consciousness become vast but dim with an in-

[26] *Integration of the Personality*, p. 15. Carl G. Jung, M. D. Translated by Stanley Dell, copyright, 1939, by Kegan Paul, and reprinted by their permission.

finite multitude of objects merging into an indistinct totality— a· state in which the subjective and objective are almost completely identical. This is all very well, but scarcely to be recommended anywhere North of the Tropic of Cancer.[27]

Professor Jung seems to conclude that the superconscious experiences are "vast but dim" without any understanding of them. Any man who has had these realizations will laugh at such conclusions. Patanjali, Swami Vivekananda, and Swami Brahmananda give just the opposite point of view. They make it clear that *samadhi,* or the superconscious state, is vivid and definite. It is indeed true that in certain superconscious states the subject, object, and their relation; the perceiver, perceived, and knowledge; and the enjoyer, enjoyed, and their relation are wholly identified. All the differences vanish in the integral unity. This happens because all the manifestations merge at that time in one Absolute Existence without differentiation of any kind. So the superconscious is not unconscious; it is full of awareness; nay, it is Consciousness Itself.

It is quite unscientific, to say the least, for a scientific man to comment on these states as "scarcely to be recommended anywhere North of the Tropic of Cancer," without his knowing them at all. We do not get such impressions in studying the experiences of Judaeo-Christian types "North of the Tropic of Cancer." Does Professor Jung remember the teachings of St. Teresa? And Meister Eckhart says:

In the soul, there is an agent of the first rank, the intellect, by means of which the soul detects and knows God. It has five properties. First, it is detached from the here and now. Second, it is *sui generis,* like nothing else. Third, it is pure and uncontaminated. . . .[28]

---

[27] *Ibid.,* p. 26.
[28] *Meister Eckhart,* trans. Raymond Bernard Blakney (New York: Harper & Brothers, 1941), p. 167.

Anyone who studies the teachings and records of the experiences of Western and Eastern mystics will never make such unscientific statements as Professor Jung. The superconscious experiences of mystics in the West are identical with those of mystics in the East. Rudolf Otto says "that mysticism is *the same* in all ages and in all places, that timeless and independent of history it has always been identical. East and West and other differences vanish here."[29] As we have already said, there may be differences in the types of experiences, not because of the East or West but because of the temperaments of the individuals. We do not agree with Dr. Jung that these experiences cannot be recommended to the West. In fact, everyone, whether Eastern or Western, must have certain realization if they are to experience the Reality. Otherwise, knowledge of God and religion, as it is expressed by Professor Jung and such others, will always remain guesswork! It is interesting to note what Rudolf Otto has to say in his book, *The Idea of the Holy.* "This mental state is perfectly *sui generis* and irreducible to any other; and therefore, like every absolutely primary and elementary datum, while it admits of being discussed, it cannot be strictly defined."[30]

There are many rationalistic thinkers in the West who express ideas similar to those of Professor Jung without studying carefully the mystic practices of both Oriental and Occidental systems, especially those of the Orient. They are also equally guilty of superficiality and an unscientific attitude of mind. We deliberately considered the opinions of Professor Jung knowing that he is interested in the study of both Eastern and Western schools of thought; yet he seems to be considerably confused, to say the least. What he says is far from the truth. There is some outward similarity between

[29] Rudolf Otto, *Mysticism East and West,* trans. Bertha L. Bracey and Richenda C. Payne (London: Macmillan, 1932), p. xv, and chap. I.
[30] Rudolf Otto, *The Idea of the Holy,* trans. John W. Harvey (London: Humphrey Milfort, Oxford University Press, 1925), p. 7.

superconscious and unconscious states yet there is a world of difference between them. An average man is completely oblivious of his unconscious state. Often the unconscious contents of the mind become the causes of abnormalities and functional ailments, although they are unknown to the person concerned. In an ordinary man the unconscious states create a great many disturbances. Moreover, as he is not aware of them he cannot recognize them as such. In the superconscious experience the whole mind is illumined. A man of superconscious experience knows all the past contents of his mind. Besides, a man cannot even enter into that state unless and until the contents of the unconscious are at first controlled and integrated and then wholly emptied. It is impossible for a man to aspire for superconscious experience until and unless both conscious and unconscious states of mind are wholly purified through intense spiritual practices. So the unconscious contents and superconscious experiences are as far apart as the two poles. One is below the development of consciousness; the other is above ordinary consciousness. One becomes an obstacle of normal life; the other is the supernormal life, far above even the so-called normal states. To identify the superconscious state with the unconscious state is to mix darkness and light. In one case man is completely oblivious of the existence of God; in the other case man is fully aware of the existence of God, nay, identified with Him.[31] Swami Vivekananda describes these states of consciousness:

First is the conscious plane, in which all work is always accompanied with the feeling of egoism. Next comes the unconscious plane, where all work is unaccompanied by the feeling of egoism. That part of mind-work which is unaccompanied with the feeling of egoism is unconscious work, and that part which is accompanied with the feeling of egoism is conscious work. In the lower animals this unconscious work is called instinct. In higher ani-

[31] *Gospel of Sri Ramakrishna*, I, 87-123.

mals, and in the highest of all animals, man, what is called conscious work, prevails.

But it does not end here. There is a still higher plane upon which the mind can work. It can go beyond consciousness. Just as unconscious work is beneath consciousness, so there is another work which is above consciousness, and which also is not accompanied with the feeling of egoism. The feeling of egoism is only on the middle plane. When the mind is above or below that line there is no feeling of "I," and yet the mind works. When the mind goes beyond this line of self-consciousness it is called *Samadhi* or super-consciousness.[32]

When we study the writings of great Christian mystics, we realize that Professor Jung's conclusions are extremely superficial and erroneous. Meister Eckhart, who is one of the greatest men of realization, says: "When one takes God as he is divine, having the reality of God within him, God sheds light on everything. Everything will taste like God and reflect him. God will shine in him all the time."[33] There are states of superconscious experience which cannot be described or related through human language as they are beyond the gross state of mind.[34] Language is limited to the realm of the empirical self which dissolves at that time. Consequently, the human mind, which is the basis of the empirical self, cannot describe them. As Swami Brahmananda says:

This *Samadhi* cannot be described. It is beyond the reach of the gross mind, beyond language. It is beyond *Asti* and *Nasti* (human calculation), beyond pleasure and pain, beyond joy and sorrow, beyond light, beyond darkness, beyond all duality. Human language is too feeble to say what that blessed state is.[35]

[32] *Works*, I, 180.
[33] *Meister Eckhart*, p. 9.
[34] *Gospel of Sri Ramakrishna*, I, 88.
[35] *Spiritual Teachings of Swami Brahmananda*, p. 126.

CHAPTER XI

Methods of Superconscious Experience

THE question arises from a scientific point of view as to whether or not the superconscious experience of an individual can be verified by other people. When we study the religious history of the world, we find that there have been a few cases in which men and women have stumbled into mystic realizations without going through discipline or training. Saul, on the way to Damascus, had the wonderful experience of Jesus, the Christ, which transformed him into St. Paul and made him a great pillar of the Church of Christ. Such cases are known in India and other parts of Asia and Europe. They are generally regarded as special manifestations and expressions of the grace of God.

The scientific person likes to know if this knowledge can be gained as we learn scientific facts. In other words, is there any method by which one can know these experiences? Our answer is that certain methods lead one to these experiences, provided one follows them strictly. It is true, however, that these methods are not like scientific laboratory experiments. In the laboratory we objectively study external phenomena which are separate from us. But in studying the facts of superconscious realization we take up an altogether different method. The systems of study and investigation are subjective. We train the mind itself. Nevertheless, these methods are scientific so far as universality and possibility of verification are concerned. Just as any scientist belonging to any country, race, or religion can make required experiments, verify the scientific facts, and arrive at the same conclusions and experiences provided he is thorough and exact; so any man belonging to any country, race, or religion can have the same type of superconscious realizations provided he is thorough and exact in the methods required; and he can verify them himself. In fact, according to some great Hindu leaders, religion really begins with *samadhi*. Swami Brahmananda was emphatic on this point and he would urge his disciples to attain to spiritual realization.[1]

It may seem that this is a rigid conception of religion. The standard will appear to be very high, almost beyond the realm of ordinary men. It may be argued that under these conditions there will not be many adherents of religion. After a little consideration we cannot help but be convinced that such a statement is true. God and experiences of God are practically unknown to an average man. To him religion means following certain doctrines and rituals or believing in God and certain great spiritual personalities. God is still an intellectual conception or belief based on books and the words of others. He is not a fact of experience. Conceptual knowledge of God and actual experience of Him are quite different; in fact, there is a world of difference between them. The effect of such experience of God, as we discussed in the previous chapter, shows that one must have superconscious realization for immediate and direct knowledge of God. Therefore, verification is the best confirmation or proof of religious experiences, and as such it is scientific. The methods are also scientific, as they lead to the realization of religious truth.

It is often argued that these experiences come to a man through divine grace and divine intervention, and we cannot do anything about them. Sometimes devout persons seem to think that it is sacrilegious even to consider adopting spir-

[1] *Spiritual Teachings of Swami Brahmananda.*

itual practices to attain the experience of God. They feel that spiritual experiences come only through divine grace, that our duty is to remain passive so that the divine will and power may function through us.

We agree that there are some such cases in the religious history of the world, when men and women have had superconscious experience of God without any effort on their part. But such cases are few and far between in both the East and the West. On the other hand, most of the great religious personalities followed systematic practices which enabled them to reach the goal of life, God-consciousness, after gradually going through the different mystical experiences. There are also other persons who disciplined themselves enough to have these high spiritual experiences and superconscious states. The Christian mystic orders of St. Bernard, St. Francis, St. Teresa, St. John of the Cross, Meister Eckhart, Thomas à Kempis, and others had definite systematic spiritual discipline and training for the realization of ordinary religious experiences. We can especially mention the mystical exercises of St. Ignatius and St. Teresa. Thomas à Kempis gives helpful suggestions for spiritual exercises.[2] The Christian mystics who really had the different types of superconscious experiences gave tremendous emphasis to spiritual practices. Also, in some of the Jewish mystic organizations certain disciplinary processes or devotional practices are advocated for superconscious realization. Some branches of Mohammedanism prescribe methods for the realization of God. Hinduism and Buddhism made scientific investigation of these experiences as well as of the methods for attaining them; and, as a result, we find well-developed scientific details in the methods for superconscious realization in the Hindu system.

[2] Thomas à Kempis, *Following of Christ* (New York: Catholic Publishing Co.), p. 549.

The teachings of Sri Krishna in the *Gita*, the teachings of Patanjali, and those of other great Hindu spiritual teachers give us various methods after studying the different temperaments of individuals. These methods are called *yogas*. This word is often grossly misunderstood in the West, especially in America. Most people seem to think that *yoga* is thought reading, fortune telling, "rope tricks," or expressions of mysterious powers. We need not say who is responsible for this erroneous interpretation of the word. However, we realize that *yoga* is a foreign word, and Americans are not likely to know its proper meaning. It really signifies "union," being derived from the root *yuj*—to yoke. Through *yoga* we are joined to God. There is no mystery mongering connected with it. Patanjali defines *yoga* as the complete control of the mind-stuff (*chitta vrittis*).[3] When the mind is fully controlled, the Truth reveals Itself. Mental calmness and tranquillity can be attained in various ways through the different *yogas*. Swami Vivekananda, the great authority on *yoga* in theory and practice, tells us:

There are various such *Yogas* or methods of union—but the chief ones are—*Karma-Yoga, Bhakti-Yoga, Raja-Yoga,* and *Jnana-Yoga.*

Every man must develop according to his own nature. As every science has its methods, so has every religion. The methods of attaining the end of religion are called *Yoga* by us, and the different forms of *Yoga* that we teach, are adapted to the different natures and temperaments of men. We classify them in the following way, under four heads:—

(1) *Karma-Yoga*—The manner in which a man realises his own divinity through works and duty.

(2) *Bhakti-Yoga*—The realisation of the divinity through devotion to, and love of, a personal God.

(3) *Raja-Yoga*—The realisation of a man's own divinity through the control of mind.

[3] *Yoga Aphorisms of Patanjali* I:2.

(4) *Jnana-Yoga*—The realisation of a man's own divinity through knowledge.

These are all different roads leading to the same centre—God.[4]

According to Hindu teachers, human minds are grouped into four distinct types: intellectual, emotional, active, and meditative. Apart from that, these different types are subdivided according to the mental structure of innumerable individuals, and every one of these types and individuals has distinct methods for spiritual development. Superconscious realizations are processes of spiritual evolution and not of superimposition, so the teachers try to find out the individual characteristics of the different aspirants and accordingly prescribe individual methods to suit their temperaments and mental capacities. However, there are common requisites for all types of minds. For instance, the science of ethics is the foundation of spiritual practices for all temperaments. Without thorough ethical training one cannot expect to have a controlled mind. The practice of ethical principles and psychology go together. According to Indian spiritual teachers, superconscious experiences are based on the science of ethics and higher psychology. As we related previously, one cannot have the power of concentration unless one tries to control and purify the mind and develop basic ethical qualities. This is what the Christian mystics call the "purgative state" and what the Hindus call *yama* and *niyama* or *shama* and *dama*. When the mind is purified it can then be focused on God. The great spiritual personalities of the world stressed this in their teachings. Jesus said: "Blessed are the pure in heart: for they shall see God."[5] Sri Krishna declares:

> But the self-controlled man, moving among objects with senses under restraint, and free from attraction and aversion, attains to tranquillity.

[4] *Works*, V, 219-20.
[5] Matt. 5:8.

In tranquillity, all sorrow is destroyed. For the intellect of him who is tranquil-minded, is soon established in firmness.

No knowledge (of the Self) has the unsteady. Nor has he meditation. To the unmeditative there is no peace. And how can one without peace have happiness?[6]

Patanjali emphasized that inner and outer purification is absolutely necessary for spiritual growth; *yama* and *niyama* are the first steps toward higher realization.[7] Sri Ramakrishna said: "God is seen when the mind is perfectly tranquil."[8] Therefore, ethical practices are a prerequisite for any method of superconscious realization. The practice of concentration can be fruitful only when the mind is made quiet through higher ethical purification and the whole nervous system is purified and strengthened through the practice of *yama* and *niyama*.

The intellectual type of seeker follows the rationalistic method of distinguishing the truth from the untruth, the real from the unreal, by using the power of discrimination and analysis. This is *Jnana Yoga*. An adamantine will power is required for this method as transitory phenomena and non-essentials have to be negated and rejected in order to know the permanent, the Absolute. The emotions must be controlled and regulated; in fact, no emotional expression should be permitted because any kind of emotional expression presupposes plurality and duality. A follower of *Jnana Yoga* must constantly remind himself of unity. Anything that arouses the consciousness of multiplicity must be completely rejected. In order to achieve this, one must develop the power of concentration and will. This method seems to be quite contrary to the ordinary functionings of human beings, as we are always giving vent to our emotions;

[6] *Srimad-Bhagavad-Gita* II:64-66.
[7] *Yoga Aphorisms of Patanjali* II:29-33, and *Vivekachudamani*.
[8] *Sayings of Sri Ramakrishna* XX:392.

moreover, our activities presuppose a certain kind of emotional background.

The practice of concentration and meditation in *Jnana Yoga* is very difficult for an average man or woman as one has to focus the mind on the "impersonal," non-bodily, Self-conscious Absolute (*Sat-chid-ananda, Nirguna Brahman*). It is very difficult for an ordinary person who is living on the plane of time-space-causal relationship and name, form, and attributes to conceive anything that is beyond these categories. It is true that certain symbols like sound and light are often given as the objects of concentration; but even such a symbol or substitute of the unconditioned Absolute (*Nirguna Brahman*) is difficult for the beginners of this path to use as an ideal. So this intellectual method is not appropriate for the average man and woman, as life on an ordinary level would become confusing. There are few persons in the world who can start their spiritual practices entirely from the intellectual point of view. They require tremendous discipline and ethical training to begin with this method. It is nice to talk of principles and philosophy; but it is altogether a different matter to practice the life of intellect; and it is still harder to see the oneness of life and existence in ordinary human behavior. In fact, a follower of *Jnana Yoga*, or the intellectual path, must try to find unity and divinity in every thought and action. He must try to find the Absolute beyond the relative. This must be the constant practice, and all activities must be regulated to it. Gradually plurality, and even duality of every type, vanishes. One has to eliminate all consciousness of difference in everyday life. So it is difficult for an ordinary person to follow this path even though he may be a philosopher. Many persons seem to think that they are Absolutists in their philosophy but their actions reveal that they are still functioning on the lower plane of relative existence, or *Maya*. According to Hindu thinkers, they are still living in ignorance.

A great American philosopher told us about a professed Absolutist in this country. We shall cite the case with due respect for the intellect of this Absolutist. It was reported that after World War I the question was raised whether or not the American Philosophical Association should resume intellectual relations with German philosophers. The Absolutist opposed the suggestion on the ground that he desired no relations with Germans. This is not a singular instance; we have seen such cases all over the world. A person may have intellectual flights of Absolutism yet, emotionally, he remains on the very common plane where hatred and other such tendencies of differentiation still function. When a man is aware of diversity and does not use his discrimination, he cannot attain knowledge of the Absolute. That is the very reason that Vedanta Aphorisms[9] teach that one must have an intense desire for higher knowledge and be ready to sacrifice everything for its attainment; that is to say, one must give up longing for anything that arouses consciousness of duality or plurality or that is a reminder of physical existence and separate consciousness. He must possess keen power of discrimination and, above all, higher ethical qualities. Then alone can one follow the path of analysis. Ethical qualities are the prerequisites of this path. It is, however, possible to take it up after a considerable amount of progress has been made through other practices.

Emotional persons have to begin with their emotions in attaining spiritual realization. They follow *Bhakti Yoga* or the path of love and devotion. The vast majority of the people in the world are predominantly emotional, so it is both convenient and necessary for them to use their emo-

---

[9] *Brahma Sutra* with Sri Sankaracharya's Commentary (Introduction) and *Vivekachudamani* by Sri Sankaracharya.

tions for higher spiritual development. We can hardly find a man or woman who has not strong emotional urges, and it is considered wise to express them instead of starving or discarding them. Emotions are great powers; a seeker after truth is, therefore, asked to direct them to an aspect of God which is suitable to his own temperament. It is not correct to assume that they can be directed to only one particular aspect of God and not to any other. Some people become narrow and bigoted in their spiritual life and insist on one aspect as the only object of love and devotion for everyone. As the All Loving Being is infinite He has infinite aspects. Psychologically speaking, human beings have different mental attitudes and degrees of power. When they try to conceive of God with the mind limited by the conditions of time-space relationship, their minds are generally limited by the reactions to the objective world of name and form. They also have certain predispositions and preconceived notions of the objects that they experience. Consequently, they have different types of emotions according to prepossessed inclinations. In fact, the mind is extremely limited to the finite conditions of life. As such, they necessarily see God with their limited mental possibilities for the time being. Therefore, there will always remain differences in the understanding of God. Hindu spiritual leaders maintain that these differences and variations do not affect the spiritual growth of an individual. On the contrary, their opinion is that in the beginning of spiritual life everyone must take a particular aspect of God suitable to his own individual inclinations and possibilities. In fact, according to them, spiritual growth is accelerated if one can take an aspect of God for meditation according to his inner nature, as we explained in the chapter on "Meditation."

It is also fallacious to think that God can be conceived only as father and not as mother, friend, beloved, or child.

All the emotions characteristic in such human relationships can be applied to God according to individual temperaments and requirements. That is the very reason the devotional mystics vary in their methods of approach to God. Some few may like to think of Him as their child, while more prefer to look on Him as father or mother, and again others will love God as their friend or beloved because this attitude is best suited to their individual temperaments and this relationship is natural and spontaneous to them. These relationships are called *bhavas* by Hindu religious leaders.[10] They are: *shanta* (placid love for the Creator, Lord, and Ruler); *dasya* (relationship between master and servant); *sakhya* (friendship between two friends); *vatsalya* (love between child and parent); and *madhura* (sweet relationship between lovers). Some devotees also establish a relationship in which God is the mother and the devotee is the child.[11] These *bhavas* should be cultivated and established almost according to the same patterns of our human behavior to our beloved ones. Many Christian mystics and others also followed this process of establishing loving relationships with God according to the predominant tendencies of their own minds. With this method, relationship with God becomes easy and effective, and at the same time the natural innate tendencies are not wasted.[12] Every person has certain spontaneous urges. Hindu teachers want their followers to use and direct their natural inclinations, for experience proves that people grow immensely in this way as they have the satisfaction of expressing their innate emotional powers. It has been found by Hindu teachers that when one cultivates such a loving relationship with God spiritual growth is accelerated. One reaches the supreme goal of life by following any of these

[10] See *Bhagavatam*; Vaishnava literature of India; Narada, *Bhakti Sutra*; and Swami Saradananda, *Sri Sri Ramakrishna Lilaprasanga*, II.

[11] *Works*, III, 92-98.

[12] *Sayings of Sri Ramakrishna*, chap. XXV.

bhavas. However, no *bhava* should be changed for another until the spiritual aspirant reaches the culmination of a relationship. A person can, however, change one relationship for another after becoming thoroughly established in the *bhava* and after experiencing the All Loving Being through it. This was done by Sri Ramakrishna.[13]

In order to cultivate emotional relationships with God, one is advised to take up various auxiliary methods, such as external and internal worship and other such practices. In external worship a devotee tries to think of God through worship with material ingredients such as flowers, light, incense, perfume, and food. With internal worship, a devotee is required to direct his emotions along with the offerings of inner qualities and attributes and elements of his body and mind. Some of the devotees also try to remember and recapitulate the incidents in the lives of Incarnations like Krishna, Buddha, and Christ. Remembrance of the Passion and other incidents in the lives of these great personalities are helpful for integrating and unifying the whole mind. Some of these aspirants often adopt the repetition of the name of God as a practice. Hindu mystics have developed a science of the repetition of the name of God (*mantra shatra*), and according to them, a seeker after truth can have the highest states of superconscious realization by repeating some of the symbolic names of God while meditating on Him at the same time. There are different short names for the various aspects of God; and, as we recorded in the chapter on "Meditation," these names vary according to the temperament of the individuals. The progress of the devotees greatly depends on the choice of these names. Repetition helps the devotees in attaining that concentration which leads their minds to the deepest state of meditation. Swami Brahmananda empha-

[13] Swami Saradananda, *Sri Sri Ramakrishna Lilaprasanga*, II.

H

sizes the importance of *japam* (repetition of the name of God):

Japam. Japam. Japam. While you work, practice *japam.* Let the wheel of the name of God go round and round in the midst of all activities. Do this! All the burning of the heart will be soothed. Don't you know how many sinners have become pure and free and divine by taking refuge in the name of God? Have intense faith in God and in His name. Know that God and His name are one. He dwells in the hearts of His devotees. Call on Him earnestly. Pray to Him: "Reveal Your grace to me. Give me faith and devotion." Pray earnestly. Make your mind and your lips one.

Cover everything with God. See Him in all creatures. As you learn to see God everywhere, you will become "humbler than a blade of grass." Hear only of God and talk only of Him. Shun that place where His name is not uttered as you would a crema-tion-ground.

.   .   .   .

Repeat His name and call on Him. He is very near and dear to all. Why should He not reveal Himself? Open your heart to Him. He will guide you along the right path. There is nothing more purifying than His name and meditation upon Him. He is our very own. He easily becomes revealed to us.[14]

Historically we find there have been many great personalities who reached the higher mystical experiences through this practice. It has been recorded that it is the easiest and the most suitable process of realizing the truth in this age. Sri Ramakrishna, the great modern Hindu leader, emphasized its value. Sir John Woodruff has translated some of the Hindu scriptures dealing with this subject.

The active types of persons can reach superconscious realization by performance of unselfish work without attach-ment. This is called *Karma Yoga.* Sri Krishna says:

[14] *The Eternal Companion*, p. 145.

The truly admirable man controls his senses by the power of his will. All his actions are disinterested. All are directed along the path to union with Brahman.

. . . .

Do your duty always; but without attachment. That is how a man reaches the ultimate truth; by working without anxiety about results.[15]

There is a technique of doing work.[16] One must forget one's self in the action and also completely forget the result that is achieved thereby. Sri Krishna tells us: "Thy right is to work only; but never to the fruits thereof."[17] In this method a devotional person constantly remembers God in and through action and an intellectual person remembers the Absolute and feels oneness in the universe. The followers of *Karma Yoga* try to see the manifestation of God in all and serve them accordingly. To them a sick man, an illiterate person, a weak individual steeped in ignorance and expressing lower tendencies is a veritable manifestation of God; and so they serve suffering humanity. They do not go out to do "charity," nor do they have the idea that they are helping these people. On the contrary, they serve them with love and devotion. Swami Vivekananda, the great champion of *Karma Yoga* in this age, says:

Look upon every man, woman and every one as God. You cannot help anyone; you can only serve: serve the children of the Lord, serve the Lord Himself, if you have the privilege. If the Lord grants that you can help any one of His children, blessed you are; do not think too much of yourselves. Blessed you are that that privilege was given to you, when others had it not. Do it only as a worship. I should see God in the poor, and it is for my salvation that I go and worship them. . . . Bold are my words,

---

[15] *Bhagavad-Gita*, trans. Swami Prabhavananda (1944), pp. 53-55.
[16] *Works*, I, 23-116.
[17] *Srimad-Bhagavad-Gita*, trans. Swami Swarupananda (1933), II:47.

and let me repeat that it is the greatest privilege in our life that we are allowed to serve the Lord in all these shapes.[18]

There are, however, persons (some of the Buddhists), who attained illumination without any thought of a personal or impersonal God by performing action for its own sake, forgetting themselves completely and remaining indifferent to the result of action.

There is a dispute as to the efficacy of this path and whether *Karma Yoga* alone can lead one to the knowledge of Reality or whether it is merely a stepping stone to higher spiritual practices. Some thinkers, even those in Hindu groups, seem to be of the opinion that the path of action should be followed for the purpose of purifying the individual; then when the person becomes fit for higher meditation and other devotional exercises, he should intensify these practices and give up action. According to these thinkers, action of any type cannot lead one directly to the Absolute. Others, again, are of the opinion that one should combine work with worship or with devotional practices and meditation. Their view is that the combination of these two methods, work and devotion (*Karma Yoga* and *Bhakti Yoga*), will lead one to the highest realization; and until this goal is reached, one must continue with the combined method. But Sri Krishna and Swami Vivekananda are clear that one can attain the goal of religion by following any one of these methods. Sri Krishna says that "only children make the distinction." That is to say no one path is superior to another. Then again he declares: ". . . the path of knowledge for the meditative, the path of work for the active."[19] He also tells us that many persons have attained perfection by following *Karma Yoga*.

We should note in connection with *Karma Yoga* that it has

---

[18] *Works*, III, 246-47.
[19] *Srimad-Bhagavad-Gita* III:3.

no place for restless activity. A *Karma Yogi* must always be alert that the mind does not get mixed up with ambition and so-called "self-expression." Like the *Jnana·Yogi* he should always try to eliminate self-consciousness or the ego. It is quite conceivable that in the midst of activities, however well meaning he may be in the beginning, the ego of a person is stimulated by the objective success of the work. However, success in *Karma Yoga* does not mean external achievement but rather inner purification and conquest of the lower self. Let there be no confusion about the process of *Karma Yoga* and achievements by that method; otherwise, it will defeat itself by merely producing external and objective results in the form of success in creating bigger and better institutions, cities, etc. If *Karma Yogis* are not careful of the inner workings of the mind in the form of ambition for external achievement, their activities will no longer remain as true *Karma Yoga*. So the path of action may not necessarily lead to success in the objective sense but rather in the subjective sense; that is to say, it should lead a person to a peaceful state of mind, as it emphasizes conquest of desire for the fruit of action. Therefore, the great spiritual leaders often advise beginners on this path to practice meditation, worship, or any other auxiliary method to keep the ideal bright and the mind free from desire for ambition and "self-expression." It is, however, possible for a few persons to follow *Karma Yoga* strictly without any auxiliary method.

We should also note that this is predominantly an age of action; and Swami Vivekananda, great teacher of all the systems of *yoga*, convincingly tells us that most of the people will have to follow the path of action more or less. In fact, the right form of action, or *Karma Yoga*, is applicable to all spiritual aspirants, and they do follow certain phases of *Karma Yoga* in the course of their spiritual evolution. Sri Krishna says in the *Gita* that man works being impelled by his very nature.[20] So it is a mistake to think that spiritual persons become other-worldly and neglect their duties in life. On the contrary, the real teachers of the systems of *yoga*, like Sri Krishna and Swami Vivekananda, glorify the active elements in man by giving them proper direction so that his activities can lead him to the direct and immediate realization of God. It goes without saying that the path of action is not just a mere step to higher practices whereby one is purified, made unselfish and otherwise fit for them; but it is a definite path in itself, leading one to the same goal that is reached by any of the other *yogas—Jnana, Bhakti,* or *Raja.*

The meditative people have to take up certain forms of concentration and meditation, as they are described in the chapter on "Meditation," to reach superconscious experience. This is *Raja Yoga* or the psychological method. The word *Raja* means "royal." The practice of concentration and meditation is needed more or less in every path in different ways, so it is regarded as a "royal" path. This psychological method helps one to integrate the mind; all mental states are unified. Moreover, a scientific man can follow it step by step and train his mind even if he cannot, for the time being, accept the idea of God. Many Buddhists and Hindus have started with this psychological *yoga* and have reached the goal. In fact, when the mind is well regulated, controlled, and unified, the truth reveals itself. The eightfold steps of *Raja Yoga* have been elaborately explained in Chapter VI. Therefore, to avoid repetition only a brief statement is made here.

Many Western and Eastern readers are often interested in *Hatha Yoga.* People frequently confuse it with *Raja Yoga* as there are some common physical steps in both. It will be interesting to note here that Hindu psychologists of the *Raja Yoga* type have found in the course of their experiences that physical health is important for mental development, as the

---

[20] *Ibid.,* III:5.

mind of the average person functions through the nervous system. When the body is sick or weak, the nervous system is consequently affected. The mind becomes restless or uncontrollable, and it also often becomes dull, inert, and sleepy. These states are obstacles to higher mental development. In order to practice the last four steps—*pratyahara* (withdrawal of the mind), *dharana* (concentration), *dhyana* (meditation), and *samadhi* (superconscious)—a person must have control over the physical functions of the body. He must also have strong nerves; otherwise he cannot have effective concentration or meditation, and it becomes impossible for him to attain the last step of *Raja Yoga*. Many of the *yogis* in the earlier days of their practice of *Raja Yoga* observe certain *Hatha Yoga* practices, which are mostly physical, in order to strengthen the physical constitution. That is one of the reasons *Raja Yoga* is sometimes regarded as a psychophysical process of the attainment of truth.

Unfortunately, it was found that many persons who practiced *Hatha Yoga* developed some of the extrasensory perceptions and occult or psychic powers, and they forgot the primary objective of *yoga* practices. These powers are regarded as obstacles (which were discussed in the chapter on "Extrasensory Experiences"), so we deliberately do not propose to give an elaborate treatment of *Hatha Yoga*, though many Western readers will be deeply interested in some of these practices for the purpose of using mental power for control of these physical laws.

Some thinkers subdivide the four main divisions of *yoga*— *Jnana, Bhakti, Karma,* and *Raja.* For instance, *Mantra Yoga* and such other subdivisions actually form parts of one of the main divisions. Outstanding leaders like Swami Vivekananda did not feel the necessity of separate treatment; they are not being mentioned separately here, as it would only create confusion.

It is difficult for beginners to get settled in higher spiritual practices. The mind remains restless; and if a person continues one form of practice, it becomes monotonous. So it is most advisable that the different methods—study, devotion, work, and meditation—be combined until a genuine interest in and love for God are created. Otherwise, there is great danger of reaction and dryness in the spiritual practices. Many persons have given up the exercises and ruined their progress because they were not wisely directed. Again, many devotees, in their early enthusiasm, try to imitate great saints and spiritually well-established persons. They try to intensify meditation or worship and ignore other aspects of life and activity, even in the beginning of religious life. They need guidance so that they will not have bad reactions, dryness, and lack of interest. So it is always desirable to have a little variation in the early stages of spiritual practices. A good thought has been expressed by a devotee: "We all have our Destination, although different paths we choose to the storehouse of Infinite Knowledge for the Self to explore."

Swami Vivekananda was the advocate of developing and harmonizing these four methods or *yogas* in the individual. He felt that, if anyone would combine two or three methods, he would have more harmonious development than otherwise. There would not be any possibility of narrowness or one-sidedness, and the character would be well rounded and fully developed. It is, however, difficult for one to perfect one's self in all of them simultaneously. There are, of course, persons who can do it, but usually one feels quite successful if he can reach the goal by following one system thoroughly. It goes without saying that one must perfect one's self in whatever method is adopted in order to attain the desired realization. However, partial practice or combination of some of the methods is extremely elevating and desirable, especially for beginners. One should be careful not to lose interest in

God by being injudicious in practices. One should also be careful in making the right choice of the methods according to one's own temperament. According to Swami Brahmananda:

All these have one and the same purpose—God realization. There is so much difference between one man and another in their inclinations and their temperaments that no one method can be assigned to all for their *Sadhana* or spiritual advancement. Different temperaments require different *Sadhana* and different ways of worship. To meet these varying demands the Scriptures have prescribed four principal means,—*Samadhi* [direct worship of the Absolute], *Dhyana* [meditation, where the worshiper remains separate], actual *Japam* [repetition of the name of God], prayer and external worship.[21]

As the different *yogas* or methods all lead one ultimately to God, so do the various creeds and religions of the world.

[21] *Spiritual Teachings of Swami Brahmananda*, p. 130.

CHAPTER XII

Can Superconscious Knowledge Be Imparted?

THERE is a legitimate question in the minds of the vast majority of scientific thinkers as to whether or not superconscious knowledge can be imparted to others. If it is to be scientifically investigated it must be communicable. Many devout religious persons are of the opinion that this knowledge comes through the grace of God, as we mentioned in the previous chapter; consequently, it cannot be the object of scientific investigation, nor can it be communicated as one person gives an object to another. The history of religion proves to us that superconscious knowledge as well as the lower extrasensory perceptions, psychic and occult powers can be transmitted and received. Of course, there are certain necessary conditions to be fulfilled by the person who communicates them and the person who receives them. In the first place, every person who stumbles into certain extraordinary experiences, whether they are occult powers or higher superconscious realizations, cannot transmit these powers to others as effectively as it is desirable. When a person stumbles into spiritual experiences, he can have certain definite realization of the Ultimate Reality. Yet because he has not developed the technique and is not well established in it he cannot transmit that knowledge directly and immediately to others. He can, perhaps, describe some of his experiences and give some idea of his personal realizations. On the other hand, when a man is thoroughly established in the superconscious, whether through certain practices or through divine grace, he can transmit this power and this knowledge to others—not as mediate knowledge but as direct perception.

It is true, however, that the exact nature of emotional reaction in certain spiritual realizations cannot be communicated and cannot be made enjoyable through oral expressions, just as the emotion of love cannot be qualitatively given to anyone. In order to understand the real effect of love, one must fall in love. A mother cannot communicate her inner emotion to anyone else. In order to understand a mother's love one has to be a mother. Similarly, spiritual realizations, whether they come almost instantly through divine intervention alone or through spiritual practice and divine intervention combined, cannot be communicated in their qualitative value, nor can they be fully described by human language as to their quantitative value, since they are unique experiences so far as the persons are concerned—just as the experience of love is unique.

It is also true that there are some systematic methods by following which one can reach these experiences. The so-called extrasensory perceptions, occult powers, and such other extraordinary display of mental or psychic powers can, of course, be expressed as prescribed by Patanjali in *Raja Yoga*. The higher superconscious realizations can also be reached by systematic methods, as Patanjali and other great religious leaders of other countries and religions prescribed, and which we studied in the last chapter.

The person who transmits or gives this knowledge is the *Guru* (teacher), and the person who receives it is the *shisya* (disciple). The *Guru* is not an ordinary teacher of the type we hear about in the church schools and other schools of the West. The conception of *Guru* is deep and significant in spiritual life. According to most of the Hindu authorities, one can hardly expect to reach the higher state of divine realization without the help of his *Guru*. Swami Brahmananda says:

> It is not so easy without a *Guru*. The *Guru* is one who shows the path of God through a *mantram* (holy name). He gives the secret of spiritual practices. He watches over his disciple and protects him from going astray. A *Guru* must be a knower of Brahman.[1]

As a *Guru* is so essential to the spiritual development of his disciples, the required qualifications of the religious teacher should be understood.

As mentioned previously, a teacher of higher psychology or spiritual realization must be thoroughly established in those experiences to teach others. His mind must be fully illumined—first, through ethical practices and next, through practices of concentration, meditation, and such other disciplinary processes. When a man is established in higher realizations, his mind becomes completely colorless or free from all preconceived notions and impressions, and he can empty the contents of his mind at will. When he tries to impart suitable methods for spiritual practices and training to his disciple, he makes his mind completely free from all preconceived thoughts and ideas; and, consequently, he can immediately understand the very nature of his disciple. He can also understand the distinct qualities of that particular mind. A *Guru* must also inspire confidence and devotion within the student; the relation between these two persons must be extremely harmonious and loving. A teacher goes through the difficulties of imparting knowledge to the disciple only because of his intense love for him. To use the modern psychological term, there must be a "transference" of the highest type between the teacher and the disciple. This relationship is created not only because of the love between

---

[1] *The Eternal Companion*, p. 184.

them but also because of the convictions of both. The teacher must have faith in his student, believing that the student is capable of learning what he is to teach. The teacher, through his deep understanding, also knows the future possibilities of the student, and his conviction and faith brings out the student's latent possibilities.[2]

The *shisya* (disciple), too, must have the necessary qualities for higher realization and development. In the first place, he must have confidence in the teacher and devotion and love for him. Then he must have the spirit of obedience and be ready to follow implicitly the advice and instructions of the teacher. This does not, however, preclude the questioning spirit. A student is always encouraged to ask questions. "Know That (Truth) by questioning" the Hindu scriptures tell us. The spirit of humility is the most important condition for spiritual development, however, although questions and inquiries are much encouraged in a real spiritual relationship between teacher and student. The student must also have perseverance and tenacity in order to continue the practices and discipline according to instructions. There are some persons who, out of curiosity, like to make a little experiment for a few days, and then they give up the practices. This fickleness of attitude has been extremely discouraged by all religious psychologists. Patanjali regards this as one of the greatest obstacles to spiritual unfoldment. Swami Vivekananda strongly emphasized *shraddha* (dynamic faith and consequent action). Without this tenacious faith and consequent perseverance in practices, a student can hardly expect to have any of the higher realizations.

It is true that often students get discouraged because they cannot reach the goal as soon as they had expected. One can easily understand that the practice for higher realizations requires tremendous patience, as we have to struggle with

[2] *Works*, IV, 19-27.

the illusive and restless mind. Unfortunately, our minds are much agitated and colored by innumerable past experiences. Apart from that, the subconscious impressions (*samskaras*), the accumulated residuals of past thoughts and actions, are so strong that they agitate the mind all the time. Modern psychoanalysts and others find it amazing to what extent the subconscious states disturb the conscious mind. Indian psychologists thoroughly understand this factor. Consequently, they warn the students not to be disturbed or discouraged when they find that it is difficult to hold the mind on the object of concentration. Swami Brahmananda gives methods by which a disciple can be helped through such difficult periods:

These are the different stages through which the aspirant progresses. A man should begin from where he stands. If, for instance, an ordinary man is told to meditate on union with the Absolute Brahman, he cannot grasp the truth of it; nor can he follow the instructions. He may make the attempt, but soon he will tire and give it up. However, if the same man is asked to worship God with flowers, perfume, and other accessories he will find that his mind gradually becomes concentrated on God and he will soon experience a joy in his worship. Through ritualistic worship, devotion to the performance of *japam* grows. The finer the mind becomes, the greater is its capacity for higher forms of worship. *Japam* inclines the mind toward meditation. Thus the aspirant moves toward his Ideal by a process of natural growth.[3]

This shows that a disciple needs careful attention in the early stages of spiritual development. The *Guru* removes difficulties of various types from the path of the disciples. However, there are "dark hours of the soul," as described by the Christian mystics; but the *Guru*, with his own spiritual insight, understands the inner struggles of his disciples and directs them accordingly. He fully realizes the pitfalls on the path

[3] *The Eternal Companion*, p. 103.

of spiritual effort and warns against such discouragement. Patanjali, Swami Vivekananda, and others say that steady practice is absolutely necessary to overcome obstacles;[4] but when the teacher is qualified and the student is fit, then the result is positive. "Wonderful is its teacher, and (equally) clever the pupil. Wonderful indeed is he who comprehends it taught by an able preceptor."[5]

A great spiritual personality who is perfectly established in higher realizations can transmit this knowledge to a disciple even if the disciple has not undergone vigorous spiritual practices. Sri Ramakrishna, who was born in 1836 in India, could transmit spiritual power and various experiences immediately and directly to his disciples. His biography contains descriptions of such occurrences.[6] Swami Vivekananda was about eighteen years old when he first went to see Sri Ramakrishna. The great Master touched the chest of the young aspirant, who at once entered into the highest state of superconscious realization immediately and directly. He lost his physical consciousness in the realization of the Ultimate Reality. One day when Swami Brahmananda was rubbing oil on the body of Sri Ramakrishna, he too entered into superconscious realization spontaneously and immediately. He not only lost the consciousness of the external and objective world but he experienced the Ultimate Reality. On another occasion, this great Master wrote a name of God on the tongue of another disciple, who then had the realization of the personal aspect of God, his chosen Deity. We know from the history of that period that this great man had a peculiar power of awakening the latent possibilities of his disciples, and that innumerable men and women had their highest realizations from him either by a touch, a word, a wish, or

[4] *Yoga Aphorisms of Patanjali* I:13.

[5] *Katha Upanishad* II:7.

[6] Romain Rolland, *The Life of Ramakrishna* (Mayavati, Almora, Himalayas: Advaita Ashrama, 1931).

even a glance. One of the greatest disciples of the Master,
Swami Shivananda, told us that all of the disciples had the
highest realization (*samadhi*) during the lifetime of the
Master. Their lives prove to us without the least shade of
doubt that they were well established in God either through
realization of the personal (bodily) aspect or through the Impersonal (formless) aspect of God. These two types of realization are mentioned by St. Paul: "I knew a man in Christ . . .
(whether in the body, I cannot tell; or whether out of the
body, I cannot tell: God knoweth)."[7]

The supremely developed person not only can transmit
this power immediately and directly to a disciple who has not
performed spiritual practices, but even the disciples of these
great teachers can awaken latent spiritual power and give the
higher realizations when they are in that particular mood.
We know definitely that Swami Vivekananda, Swami Brahmananda, and others transmitted this power on certain occasions to their disciples and devotees. It is explained by the
religious psychologists of India that still lesser personalities
can also help their disciples in awakening spiritual consciousness, provided they themselves are established in higher
realizations and the students practice according to their
advice and directions.

Two important and significant questions will arise in the
minds of many sincere persons. (1) Can a man belonging to
any religion or nationality practice *yoga*? (2) Can anyone
have superconscious experiences? These questions have various implications. We know that different religious groups
make exclusive claims for their teachings. They not only say
that their general religion itself is the only way, but they also
emphasize that one can reach God only through their own
particular denomination, religious attitude, school of
thought, or church. We shall quote Sri Ramakrishna, the

[7] II Cor. 12:2.

greatest modern spiritual leader of India, to clarify this point. Then we can answer the real questions. He says:

Different creeds are but different paths to reach the one God. Various and different are the ways that lead to the temple of Mother. . . . Similarly, various are the ways that lead to the house of the Lord. Every religion is nothing but one of such paths that lead men to God.

As with one and the same substance, gold, various ornaments are made having different names and forms, so one and the same God is worshipped in different countries and ages under different names and forms. . . .[8]

This shows that there are many paths suitable to different types of people. Knowing this fundamental fact, we can definitely reply to the first question that *yogas* can be practiced by anyone belonging to any religion or race. There is no exclusiveness in religion. As previously explained, *yoga* is the practical system for the realization of God. As such, anyone desirous of God can and must practice certain exercises. These practices are the different forms of *yoga*, which have already been described.

Theological differences in the conception of God do not affect the practice of *yoga*. Anyone belonging to any religious group with any conception of God can practice it and be helped immensely thereby. One can adapt the practices to his personal theological interpretation of the Truth. Whether or not a person is qualified depends entirely on the intensity of his desire to grow in spirituality, regardless of religious affiliations. In other words, a Hindu, Christian, Jew, Buddhist, or a Mohammedan is equally qualified if he has an intense desire to live a spiritual life.

The answer to the second question is similar to that of the first. Superconscious experiences are not the exclusive claim

[8] *Sayings of Sri Ramakrishna* XXXVIII:716 and 717.

of any particular religion or group, although some may so express. Anyone belonging to any religion can reach the goal of religious life if he systematically and thoroughly practices *yoga* or a form of real spiritual exercises, whether they are prescribed by a Hindu, Christian, Jewish, Buddhist, or a Mohammedan teacher. The religious history of the world proves to us that every one of the great religions produced many men and women of superconscious realization. It is true that there is a difference in their experiences, as we discussed in the previous chapter. It is not because of their racial, geographical, or religious affiliations that they vary, but because of their temperaments and intensity. This difference is also observed in people belonging to the same religion and even in the disciples of the same master, owing to temperamental diversities.

CHAPTER XIII

Religion and Psychotherapy

THERE is considerable dispute among many persons as to whether or not religion can contribute anything toward the stable working of the human mind. There are many others, however, who feel that psychological training is absolutely necessary for the progressive ministers of religion so that they will be able to help the unhappy conditions of their people. Let us consider the origin of mental disturbances to determine if religion, properly understood and practiced, can stabilize the minds of men and lead to real satisfaction and happiness in life.

When we study the disturbed states of the people, we recognize three different types of functional ailments: (1) neurosis, which originates in actual physical disorder such as defective brain matter and nervous system; (2) psychogenic neurosis, which originates in mental disturbances of such types as mental conflict, frustration, and discontent; and (3) psychosis, which is mental illness.

Neurosis of purely physical origin can be treated and helped medically by the neurologists. It requires technical knowledge to help neurotic conditions of this type, and only the medical authorities can be of service to such persons, as they know the structure and functioning of the nervous system and other parts of the body.

The psychogenic neurotic conditions originate in a different source. The mental conflicts and confusion are due to either abnormal primary or secondary urges. The physical side can be helped only by the neurologists or psychotherapeutists and physicians, but such treatment cannot be beneficial unless it is supplemented by a sound and satisfactory philosophy of life. This can only be given by a man who has it himself, whether he is a religious man, psychiatrist, psychologist, or a physician. Then, and then alone, can he be of service to a person who has a psychogenic neurosis. We do not like to limit religious leadership to the people who have adopted religious life. A physician or a psychologist may be equally religious if he has the proper understanding and appreciation of religious philosophy and practices. Professor Jung agrees that higher values of life can be given to a person only by a man who has them himself, and not otherwise. When we were talking together one day about the utility of the practice of concentration, he fully appreciated this view saying: "I cannot help my neighbors to keep their gardens in proper order unless I keep my own garden in order." It is of vital importance in mental training. One may be able to teach practical sciences without integrating one's own mind, but one cannot teach religion and mental culture without being established in them.

The cases of psychosis can also be immensely helped by a man of stable mind and sound philosophy. Psychosis is generated by the conflicts, confusion, and frustration of the mind and by uncontrolled emotions. Those tendencies can hardly be removed unless higher values are absorbed by the person and then practically applied in his life. When a man has the religious ideal and regulates all his activities by it, he has a satisfactory way of life. He may fail many times to reach the goal, yet the very attempt gives a great deal of satisfaction and joy to the mind. In the early stages of the struggle the conflicting elements may remain strong and cause a little disgust and disappointment, but in the long run his whole mind becomes unified because his activities are subordinated to the highest value or goal of life.

There is, however, apprehension among some of the outstanding thinkers that often religious zeal for salvation creates conflicts. But a proper philosophy of life cannot create any conflict. However sinful a man may be, however deplorable his conduct may be, he always has the possibility of redemption and enlightenment. In the teachings of Christ, St. Paul, the great Jewish mystics, and the Hindu and Buddhist leaders, we find definite understanding of the possibility of human change and transformation. A proper understanding of religion and religious ideals cannot hypnotize a man into a paralytic state nor can it create an abnormal sense of fear. On the other hand, it gives encouragement, determination, and power to reach the desired goal. Weaknesses are to be understood properly so that a man can make attempts to overcome them and have satisfaction thereby. There is great joy in the struggle of overcoming all obstacles and weaknesses. There is also joy in achieving success in the process of higher evolution.

Another concern among outstanding thinkers is that an unfavorable environment is responsible for mental conflicts. It is true that environmental conditions may create certain situations which are not conducive to the healthy growth of mental life and spiritual evolution. Yet poverty and mental disturbances are not simultaneous nor are they coexistent in certain parts of the world. A man may be poor and still have a sound philosophy of life, practicing the highest principles of ethics and religion in his everyday life. A man of humble economic condition need not necessarily be immoral or mentally restless. We find many persons of humble circumstances who possess deep spiritual qualities and mental stability in some of the Oriental countries because of their sound philosophy of life and its practical application. We know many noble souls in India who became great personalities in spite of their poverty.

Ancient and modern spiritual leaders, through their lives and teachings, remove all conflicts and frustration of the people and give a sound basis for real happiness. These principles have kept the people of India as well as early Christian civilizations peaceful and harmonious. Mental and functional diseases have been seldom found in them. We also observe that not only these great religious leaders but also some of their followers, who really organized their lives on a spiritual basis, have been the happiest persons of the world. Their lives prove to us, without the least shadow of doubt, that conflicts and frustration can be completely dissolved by the practice of spiritual philosophy in everyday living.

Sri Ramakrishna and other ancient and modern Hindu teachers tell us that God is Bliss. Anyone who meditates on Bliss, or God, gets unbounded joy. Swami Brahmananda tells us:

Try to steady it [the mind] again and again, by fixing it on the Chosen Ideal, and at last you will become absorbed in Him. If you continue your practice for two or three years, you will begin to feel unspeakable joy and the mind will become steady. In the beginning the practice of *japam* and meditation seems dry. It's like taking bitter medicine. You must forcibly pour the thought of God into your mind. As you persist you will be flooded with joy.[1]

When the poisonous element of hedonism is changed into a spiritual philosophy, the chronic symptoms of modern unhappiness in various spheres of existence automatically vanish. All the progressive laws of social security and other insurances are noble attempts to make people happy and secure but they will become meaningless if the basic phi-

---

[1] *The Eternal Companion*, p. 175.

losophy of life is not changed. It seems to us that they are doing everything to cook a good dish but are omitting the salt. All attempts to achieve good cooking become failures if the main seasoning is not given. Similarly, all the progressive laws and regulations are bound to be failures in no time if man's inner nature is not changed. If the lawmakers and administrators of law remain the same, then the beneficiaries of the laws will also remain the same. Consequently, conflicts of various types will inevitably exist; the condition of the people may be affected, but the causes will remain operative, resulting in similar difficulties. Thus, in spite of progressive thinking, we will enter into a vicious circle because of the failure to understand the root cause of the disease in modern society. All the noble attempts of modern psychiatrists will also be failures in spite of their success in certain ways. They are, no doubt, helping mankind in the Western Hemisphere to some extent, but they are only temporarily ameliorating the suffering. The real removal of the disease can only take place when psychiatry and religion in the broadest sense of the term, amalgamate, co-operate, and co-ordinate properly. Herein we find the utility of religion.

We know that there is skepticism and a critical attitude on the part of some of the psychologists and psychiatrists regarding the value of religion in psychotherapy. It is, however, conceivable that they have justification for some of their criticism regarding certain religious attitudes and interpretations of life. If we forget the creedal and ritualistic difference and go back to the teachings of the great founders of religion, we will find that there can be no two opinions regarding the value of the religious conception of life. Men differ in ritualism, ceremonies, and the use of symbols and forms. But these are not the essential part of religion. The essential part of religion emphasizes the understanding of the higher self, or God, or over soul, and the control of the lower

self or empirical self, the selfish egocentric self. Rituals, ceremonies, creeds, doctrines, and dogmas are the secondary
part of religion. If anyone imagines that religious duties are
fulfilled when he observes certain rituals and ceremonies and
has only a belief in some personalities, then, of course, psychiatrists or psychotherapeutists will have justification in
their criticism. On the contrary Sri Ramakrishna says:

> Knowledge leads to unity, but Ignorance to diversity.
> So long as God seems to be outside and far away, there is
> ignorance. But when God is realised within, that is true knowl-
> edge.
> Meditate upon the Knowledge and Bliss Eternal, and you will
> also have bliss. The Bliss indeed is eternal, only it is covered and
> obscured by ignorance. The less your attachment is towards the
> senses, the more will be your love towards God.
> Those who wish to attain God and progress in religious devo-
> tion, should particularly guard themselves against the snares of
> lust and wealth. Otherwise they can never attain perfection.
> The sun can give heat and light to the whole world, but it can
> do nothing when the clouds shut out its rays. Similarly, so long
> as egoism is in the heart, God cannot shine upon it.
> Iron, after it is converted into gold by the touch of the philos-
> opher's stone, may be kept under the ground or thrown into a
> rubbish heap; it will always remain gold and will not return to
> its former condition. Similar is the state of the man whose soul
> has touched even once the feet of the Almighty Lord. Whether
> he dwells in the bustle of the world, or in the solitude of the
> forest, nothing ever contaminates him.[2]

We need to understand that religion brings out the best
in man by manifesting the divinity that is already in him.
In fact, the higher interpretation of any religion is to bring
out the best in man. Swami Vivekananda defines religion as

[2] *Sayings of Sri Ramakrishna* I:1, 33, and 38; XXI:399; XXII:460; and
XXVII:565.

the "manifestation of the divinity that is already in man."
If we understand religion properly, we cannot help thinking
that religion alone can solve the basic problem of mental
ailments. When religious practices, creeds, rituals, ceremonies, symbols, and statues help us to manifest the divinity
in us, we then realize the goal of life. We attain joint heir-
ship with Christ, as St. Paul emphasizes in one of his
Epistles: ". . . We are the children of God: and if children,
then heirs; heirs of God, and joint heirs with Christ."[3]
Knowing this fact, we are compelled to think that when a
man tries to manifest the best in him, the divine nature in
him, the spirit of God in him, he cannot submit to his lower
passions and lower desires and aspirations.

The duty of religious leaders is to bring out the higher
qualities and not to emphasize ignoble tendencies or frighten
one because of his weaknesses. Religion is to help man remove the cause of conflict and frustration by the positive
method of revealing the divinity (*Atma*) within him. This
Reality is changeless, eternal, pure, and blissful. It has been
the experience of many scientific observers that the religious
schools which emphasize the weakness and sinful nature of
man often become the sources of discouragement, frustration, and mental conflict, as many thinkers suspect. We are
thoroughly convinced that right understanding of the religious philosophy of life, as prescribed and lived by the great
founders of religion and their successful followers, can create
no objection for psychotherapeutists. So we say that a broad
and clear understanding of religion can certainly be co-
ordinated with the technical knowledge of modern psychotherapy. In fact, psychotherapy, as practiced by psychiatrists,
and religious philosophy must go together. There is no
reason for the conflict between real religious leadership and

[3] Rom. 8:16 and 17.

real psychotherapy.[4] We are pleased to quote Professor Gordon W. Allport:

By and large psychology has done little to give systematic setting to all these various dynamic formations that represent the apex of development in the mature personality. With time, no doubt, when the errors of excessive elementarism and geneticism are cleared away, and the principle of functional autonomy is substituted as a general guide, the situation will improve.[5]

It is known to us that some of the religious leaders are rather critical and suspicious of the methods of psychotherapy. There is, unfortunately, mutual suspicion and skepticism on the part of both groups in the Western countries, but this can be removed by the proper understanding of religion. Then modern psychology would not be antagonistic to a broad interpretation of religion, nor would religion term psychotherapy an offshoot of the materialistic philosophy of life. It is true that many of the psychiatrists and psychologists in the West are materialistic in the broad sense of the term. But our contention is that if psychology is pushed beyond the physiological side, or "near-mind"[6] as Professor Hocking calls it, then psychologists will understand the reality behind the three changeable states of consciousness—waking, dreaming, and sound sleep, or conscious and subconscious.

An analysis of these three states of consciousness will convince us that there is a permanent reality behind them. In fact, that reality is the background of these three states; that *Atma*, the divine presence in man, is the substratum of them all. The very idea of these three changeable states

---

[4] Jung, *Psychology and Religion;* and *Modern Man in Search of a Soul,* chap. XXXI.

[5] Allport, *Personality, A Psychological Interpretation,* p. 227.

[6] Hocking, *Proceedings of the Sixth International Congress of Philosophy* (1927), pp. 203 and 215.

arises from the nonchangeable and permanent existence behind them. Psychology properly evolved and developed cannot help accepting a permanent reality behind the observ-
able states of consciousness. This is the fourth and it is called
turiya, the superconscious.

So it seems to us that psychology and religion properly
understood and developed to their logical conclusions will
mingle together. In fact, in India psychology is the basic
science of spiritual evolution. Religious leaders are also
ethical and psychological leaders. It is evident to us that a
man cannot become a thoroughly religious person unless
he is established in the higher principles of ethics and
psychology. He must have a thorough knowledge of and control over his mental states and thought processes in order to
have higher spiritual experiences, which were described in
previous chapters.

On the other hand, a psychologist must also have full control over his own mind in order to be effective in treating
his clients, for a man who has not integrated his own mind
cannot help in the integration of the minds of others. Professor Jung and some other psychologists fully realize that
unless a psychologist is established in his own integration
and unification of mind, having dissolved his own conflicts
and frustrations, he cannot be of any definite use to his
clients and students. It must be admitted, however, that
modern psychotherapy is ameliorating the suffering of many
persons. We make bold to say that this will serve only as a
temporary help if a higher religious background is not
furnished in removing the cause of disturbance. This means
that psychological theory alone cannot make one a psychiatrist. He must also apply the psychological principles in his
own personal life. This leads us to the conclusion that a psychotherapeutist must be a religious man in the broader sense
of the term. He may differ from others in his conception of

God. He may also differ in the methods of integration of his emotions, thought, and will according to his own natural tendencies and aptitudes. This broad principle is applicable in the higher phases of religion. Therefore, a good practicing psychotherapeutist and a good religious leader should have mental peace and happiness in common. From the Hindu point of view, psychology and religion can never be antagonistic; rather they are the two phases of the same branch of knowledge.

Both religious leaders and psychiatrists should work together for the elimination of mental disorder and conflicts. By their lives they should inspire the average man and woman. Religious leadership should furnish the philosophy or way of life and show the practical application of that philosophy in everyday living by subordinating all activities to the ideal; while psychiatrists and psychologists should furnish their technical knowledge and its application in individual cases. Of course, the persons who have organic neurosis or who have psychosis due to organic troubles should be handled entirely by the psychologists and neurologists of technical and medical knowledge, while the religious leaders should always be prepared to be of service to both the psychiatrists and the clients.

CHAPTER XIV

Philosophy of Life

MANY thoughtful persons are distressed when they observe the condition of the mental health of modern men and women. In fact, the systems of Freud, Jung, Adler, and others prove to us that these great thinkers have been extremely concerned about the mental condition of the people. When we study the statistical reports of the hospitals, we find that most of the cases can be classified into two groups: actual mental cases and functional disorders. The functional elements are really created by the maladjustment of mind which may have different emotional disturbances, complexes, dissatisfactions, and frustrations that react on the whole nervous system and result in nerve ailments and disorders. Modern psychiatrists are trying to find a remedy for removing the conflicts and frustrations and establishing harmony in the mind. Noble attempts are being made by outstanding psychiatrists of Europe and America to solve the mental problems of the people.

It is often asked whether or not religious leaders can be of any service in restoring the mental health of the people. Some of the psychiatrists seem to feel that the type of religion which is known to them does positive harm to mental health. An investigation was conducted by Professor J. McVicker Hunt of Brown University which revealed unfortunate factors in the lives of some of the mental cases of a prominent hospital in this country, as a result of emphasis on negative rather than positive qualities in man.[1] Other psychiatrists seem to feel that religion itself becomes a factor in creating conflict in the mind. As we related in the first and preceding chapters, many Freudians criticize religion for the mental harm they say it has caused. Their contention is that the mind cannot have natural expression of primitive urges because of religious fear, and so conflict is created and continues until the breaking point is reached.

We also observe that many of the Western psychologists try to solve the problem of conflict and frustration by keeping to the old hedonistic or pleasure theory of life. They seem to take it for granted that the primary objective of life is the greatest pleasure of the individual on the sense plane. Freud, in his book, *Beyond the Pleasure Principle*, discusses the pleasure and death instincts and he says: "I cannot believe in the existence of such [an impulse toward perfection] and I see no way of preserving the pleasing illusion."[2] In the same chapter he gives confusing ideas, to say the least, and shows practically no hope for human stability as he says: "Substitution or reaction formations and sublimations avail nothing toward relaxing the continual tension."[3] He and his followers do not seem to give a sound philosophy for removing difficulties, conflicts, and frustrations from human minds. Even when some advocates of the humanistic principle consider "the greatest happiness of the greatest number," the primary emphasis is given to the greatest pleasure of the individual concerned.

We cannot understand how a person can remove conflicts and frustrations by fostering hedonistic philosophy. It seems to us that frustration is inevitable so long as pleasure

[1] J. McV. Hunt, "Social Conflict in Psychosis," *The American Journal of Orthopsychiatry*, VIII (January, 1938).

[2] Sigmund Freud, *Beyond the Pleasure Principle* (London: International Psychoanalytic Press, 1922), p. 52.

[3] *Ibid.*, p. 53.

remains the primary objective of life. After all, this pleasure is limited to the sense plane. When we analyze it, we find that it is achieved in its greatest quantity when the senses are in harmonious contact with the sense objects. This harmonious contact will inevitably vary according to the changes in life; by their very nature they are changeable and impermanent.[4] The child has certain attitudes of enjoyment which change when it enters adolescence. Then again, the enjoyments of adolescents are not the same as those of adults. Grown-up and middle-aged persons cannot have the same types of pleasure as when their bodies were vigorous and strong, so their interests become different. These stages of life are inevitable, however we may dislike them. On the other hand, sense objects also change. We like to be with a particular friend, but when he changes we cease to like him. Often we find that the very person who once inspired our happiness becomes repulsive to us. Variations are inevitable both in those who enjoy the sense objects and in the objects themselves. Conditions of life and environments also change. The people who cannot adjust themselves to the variable conditions of life are bound to be full of conflicts and frustration; they are bound to be unhappy. This is especially true when they have a philosophy which emphasizes only the pleasurable aspects of life in the objective realm. Conflicts created by sense impulse or self-expression will become extremely disturbing if one persists in using these expressions only as the objective of happiness. Professor Jung in his book, *Modern Man in Search of a Soul*, aptly ridicules the women who like to be called "younger sisters of their daughters." However, we can see why mature persons would want to imitate their daughters if the primary objective of life is the greatest amount of pleasure on the sense plane. It seems to us that those unnatural ways of expression are in-

[4] *Srimad-Bhagavad-Gita* II:14.

evitable if one persists in the hedonistic point of view of life. So to our mind it is impossible for any kind of psychology to be effective and of permanent value in any society or nation, if that psychology does not change the philosophy of life. Therefore, as long as man seeks only pleasure on the sense plane as the primary objective of life, there are bound to be mental disturbances and ailments of the modern type. The mind will remain dissatisfied and unhappy, resulting in the various kinds of mental and physical ailments which we observe in the West.

We may be challenged for our evaluation of the modern Western outlook of life. Some may contend that we are underestimating this civilization. They are likely to say that religious people are generally other-worldly and, consequently, they unjustly criticize the present system of life. Let us consider the situation carefully from a comprehensive point of view.

Every civilization and every society has an *ideal* for which it works. All the activities are regulated in a way that the ideal may be expressed and fulfilled in and through the individuals and institutions of that particular society. Social, economic, political, and even religious systems are planned to fulfill that purpose. It may seem strange that we say even religion is used for expression of a collective ideal, but critical and unbiased observation of modern society will prove this to be true. The educational systems are also conditioned by that ideal; in fact, a man's whole life is expressed for its manifestation.

An individual also forms an ideal for which he works. He regulates his activities in order to express his primary objective of life and he prepares himself for that goal, whatever it may be. A person may have one of various ideals to integrate himself or his society. Eduard Spranger of Germany, and some other thinkers belonging to that school, enumerate the ideals that are taken up by the people. He tells us that there are six types: theoretical, economic, esthetic, social, political, and religious.[5] (1) A theoretical type of man takes the ideal of knowledge and truth. His supreme interest is to seek knowledge and truth in every aspect of his life. He directs his attention to philosophy, ethics, and pure science and he tries to regulate his life accordingly. (2) The economic man's aim is to fulfill the physical needs of life. He is practical in his economic adjustment, accumulation of wealth, and its use for pleasure on the sense plane. His sole aim is pleasure, and his education and even religion are used for that purpose. (It is interesting to note that universities and schools have only one aim and that is to make man fit for the sole purpose of economic security and power.) (3) The esthetic ideal inspires a man to find beauty. To him the beautiful is true and real. A poet and an artist find the expression of life in the esthetic ideal, and their lives are regulated accordingly. (4) The social ideal of man directs him to improve the social conditions of life. He considers the welfare of man. He is unselfish and sympathetic and expresses these tendencies in and through his everyday life. (5) The political man aims at the manifestation of power. His sole objective is in the political functioning of life. His interest in his fellow beings is based on an egocentric attitude, and all his activities are regulated by the urge of power. (6) The religious ideal inspires a man to find God. Unity and harmony are the objectives of his life. His activities are directed toward the fulfillment of unity in the highest sense of the term. He also prepares himself for that ideal.

When we study these six ideals of Spranger carefully, we can classify them in two groups: religious and hedonistic. Of course, there may be differences in the emphasis and application of the ideals in life, but it seems to us that the

[5] Eduard Spranger, *Types of Man* (New York: G. E. Stechert & Co., 1928).

I

mainsprings of action can be traced to either religious under-standing or pleasure on the sense plane. Economic and po-litical ideals are directly on the sense plane, while religious types mean seeking unity on the spiritual plane. Esthetic, social, and theoretical types may turn to either side as they flourish in cultures which are either sensual or religious.

Modern Western society directs its activities mainly on the sense plane. Since the Renaissance, the West has achieved wonderful results by the use of positive and applied science based on hedonism; but it has also created the cause of all the contemporary troubles in individual and collective life. There is no need for clarification; present evidences make the statement only too obvious. The conditions of present society, the structure of the family, and the life of the in-dividual would convince even a child of the validity of this statement. Professor Pitirim A. Sorokin in his masterly work, *The Crisis of Our Age,* calls the present Western civilization "sensate," while a religious society is "ideational." He also finds an "idealistic" civilization in which both are blended with "reason."

Individuals are affected by the philosophy which a society holds as an ideal. Of course, it is true that a civilization is originally built upon the ideal that is chosen by the strong personalities of that group. The present system of the West happens to be "sensate." We need not discuss how it took this turn; but we know that all activities are regulated by this ideal. It is interesting to note that even social principles, science of psychology, and other such branches of knowledge and institutions aim at that one objective. We have shown that "action" psychology expresses the inherent tendency of the sensate outlook on life; man's intelligence is evaluated by his capabilities for action. We observe that the great educationalists are emphasizing technology and applied sciences more and more, as they know that they can achieve the highest good of their ideal in that way; and thereby they can give the greatest pleasure to the people on the sense plane. We are afraid that the universities are being converted into great technological institutions instead of centers of culture for the head and heart. This is inevitable where sense pleasures are chosen as the goal of life. The result is equally axiomatic. Any farsighted man can easily predict future conditions after observing the major trend of thought in a society. Swami Vivekananda predicted the present crisis about fifty years ago. The great Swami says:

In the West, they are trying to solve the problem how much a man can possess, and we are trying here to solve the problem on how little a man can live. This struggle and this difference will still go on for some centuries. But if history has any truth in it, and if prognostications ever prove true, it must be that those who train themselves to live on the least and control themselves well, will in the end gain the battle, and that those who run after enjoyment and luxury, however vigorous they may seem for the moment, will have to die and become annihilated.[6]

Hedonism, however modified and qualified, cannot solve the problems of modern life. It is true that noble attempts in this field were made by Auguste Comte and such other humanists. There have been attempts by Karl Marx and his followers to ward off the evils that are produced by basic hedonistic philosophy and its results. It is clear that the pleasure theory of life rationalizes selfishness, greed, and love of power and position. This point of view has created great frustration both individually and collectively. A survey of historical events will reveal to us that the whole trouble with modern life arises in a wrong outlook and wrong philosophy. The great high priests of the French Revolution and the Marxian philosophers meant well in prescribing certain

[6] *Works*, III, 181.

remedies for modern evils, but it is also equally evident that their treatment of modern disease is symptomatic and like patchwork. An economic readjustment and equal distribution of the commodities of life cannot be achieved on the basis of the doctrine that pleasure is the chief good in life. The utilitarian philosophy of the greatest pleasure for the greatest number sounds very well, yet it doesn't give any real basis for a man to sacrifice his pleasure for the happiness of another.

Superficial thinkers can find a certain kind of remedy in humanism and Marxian and utilitarian philosophy for existing inequality. They may temporarily remedy certain economic and social evils, but they cannot reach the life of man. Unless his inner life is changed, conflicts and frustration will always remain. We have to consider that if we base our lives on the sense plane and make it all in all there will be inevitable frustration and disappointment, as we have already explained. The remedies that are prescribed by such thinkers, however well-meaning they are, seem to be extremely superficial and shortsighted. It seems that these thinkers are acting like shortsighted physicians who try to cure a chronic case of rheumatism by removing the pain from the ankle to the knee and from the knee to the elbow. Chronic rheumatism cannot be removed completely and thoroughly unless the cause is removed from the blood stream, which must be purified in order to be free from the various symptoms of rheumatism. However noble the attempt may be to remove the pain from the ankle or the knee, it will persist until the fundamental cause is altogether eliminated from the system. Similarly, we cannot remove the chronic rheumatism of unhappiness, mental conflicts, and frustration so long as the poisonous philosophy of life, pleasure on the sense plane, remains the ultimate objective of life. That is the very reason Swami Vivekananda advocated what he called root and branch reform. That is to say, he did not approve the symptomatic treatment of superficial thinkers; and he wanted to introduce a complete change of philosophy from hedonism to the manifestation of divinity in man, with *Paramartha* as the supreme goal of life.

We quote Professor Sorokin:

We have seen that modern sensate culture emerged with a major belief that true reality and true value were mainly or exclusively sensory. Anything that was supersensory was either doubtful as a reality or fictitious as a value. It either did not exist or, being unperceivable by the senses, amounted to the nonexistent. Respectively, the organs of senses, with the secondary help of human reason, were made the main arbiter of the true and false, of the real and unreal, and of the valuable and valueless. Any charismatic-supersensory and superrational revelation, any mystic experience, any truth of faith, began to be denied, as a valid experience, a valid truth, and a genuine value. *The major premise of the sensory nature of the true reality and value is the root from which developed the tree of our sensate culture with its splendid as well as its poisonous fruit. Its first positive fruit is an unprecedented development of the natural sciences and technological inventions.* The first poisonous fruit is a *fatal narrowing of the realm of the true reality and true value.*[7]

The learned professor gives a solution:

. . . the concerted preparation for the shift implies *the deepest reexamination of the main premises and values of sensate culture, rejection of its superannuated pseudo-values and reenthronement of the real values it has discarded.* The general line of such a reexamination and reevaluation lies in the direction of the integralist conception of truth, reality, . . . From *the integralist standpoint, the present antagonism between science, religion, philosophy, ethics, and art is unnecessary, not to mention dis-*

<hr>

[7] Pitirim A. Sorokin, *The Crisis of Our Age* (New York: E. P. Dutton & Co., Inc., 1941), p. 311.

*astrous. In the light of an adequate theory of true reality and
value, they all are one and all serve one purpose: the unfolding
of the Absolute in the relative empirical world, to the greater
nobility of Man and to the greater glory of God. As such they
should and can cooperate in the fulfillment of this greatest task.*

.   .   .   .

*Our remedy demands a complete change of the contemporary
mentality, a fundamental transformation of our system of values,
and the profoundest modification of our conduct toward other
men, cultural values, and the world at large.*[8]

So society and individuals must change their outlook.
Hedonistic philosophy will completely rob a man of what he
really seeks—happiness. He wholly defeats this primary
purpose of his life by hedonism, as we observe. The philosophy of history convinces us that the only way out is to
change the present attitude of life and establish the religious
ideal. All the religious leaders ancient and modern—the
great founders of religion like Christ, Buddha, Krishna, and
Sri Ramakrishna, as well as their followers—emphasized the
attainment of peace and happiness on the divine plane. We
read in the *Upanishads*: *"Yo vai vhuma tat sukham nalpe
sukhamasti."* "The Infinite is bliss; there is no bliss in what
is small (finite)."[9] Jesus says: "For what shall a man be
profited, if he shall gain the whole world, and forfeit his
soul? Or what shall a man give in exchange for his soul?"[10]
And St. Paul says: "For to be carnally minded is death, but
to be spiritually minded is life and peace."[11] According to
Buddha: "The gift of religion exceeds all gifts; the sweetness of religion exceeds all sweetness; the delight of religion
exceeds all delight; the extinction of thirst overcomes all

[8] *Ibid.*, pp., 316-21.
[9] *Chhandogya Upanishad*, chap. VII, sec. 23.
[10] Matt. 16:26.
[11] Rom. 8:6.

things."[12] Sri Krishna repeatedly emphasizes in the *Gita* that abiding happiness can only be reached by knowing the Self, or God, and making the activities of life on this plane of ours subordinate to the achievement of permanent knowledge of the reality of God. He declares: "That man who lives devoid of longing, abandoning all desires, without the sense of 'I' and 'mine,' he attains to peace."[13] Similarly, Sri Ramakrishna challenges the whole modern outlook of life, the pleasure theory, and declares that "the soul that has tasted the sweetness of divine bliss finds no happiness in the common pleasures of the world."[14] Swami Vivekananda's advice to the people of India is applicable to the whole world today; in fact, the world is one. Every nation and every individual is more or less affected by the present outlook of hedonism. Says the great Swami:

And, therefore, if you succeed in the attempt to throw off your religion and take up either politics or society, or any other thing as your centre, as the vitality of your national life, the result will be, that you will become extinct. To prevent this you must make all and everything work through that vitality of your religion. Let all your nerves vibrate through the backbone of your religion.[15]

Let us now be specific as to what we mean by a "religious" view of life. The Hindu view, which is for that matter the religious view, is to make the spiritual goal (*Paramartha*) the primary objective of human life. It means that man's supreme objective is to realize his divine nature (*Atma*), as we have already said. We are again reminding ourselves that "religion is the manifestation of divinity in man," as Swami Vivekananda declares. All other effort in life must be sub-

---

[12] *Dhammapada (Sayings of Buddha)*, chap. XIV.
[13] *Srimad-Bhagavad-Gita* II:71.
[14] *Sayings of Sri Ramakrishna* XXXI:603.
[15] *Works*, III, 220.

ordinated to that supreme goal. Let not anyone think that we are trying to ignore the existence of man's other cravings and that we want to create a utopian world and deny human cravings in the real world. We are not "dreamers" and "visionaries" as people often say, nor are we other-worldly. What we mean is that all activities on this relative plane must be subordinated to that supreme goal of life, instead of making the accumulation of money, supremacy over others, and the greatest pleasure the ultimate objectives. Let us not have all the functions of a man subservient to these pleasures.

We all admit that man has a desire to be happy in this sense world in various ways. He has access to the storehouse of nature and he naturally wants to use and enjoy it physically in every possible way. He wants to utilize all the forces of nature for his own comforts. His artistic and esthetic nature must be satisfied and his poetic and intellectual powers fulfilled. His emotional life has to be satisfied and harmonized. Otherwise there will be frustration and conflict. Consequently, the mind will remain an arena of disturbing urges. Man also needs proper training and equipment in order to gratify all his aspirations and hopes, desires and ambitions. We do not mean that they are to be crushed and repressed in order to follow the religious point of view. No religious leader—either of Hindu, Christian, or any other type—will ignore the facts of existence. What we suggest is to remember that those aspirations and drives must be allowed to have expression in harmony with the religious ideal. In other words, they should be expressed in such a way that we can reach the goal by utilizing them. Let not their expressions be obstacles and hindrances to the fulfillment of life. Let these desires and urges be handmaids of religious unfoldment. Let them be helpful to religious development toward the supreme goal (Paramartha).

We need proper equipment and practical training for the enjoyment of physical, intellectual, and esthetic expressions. This training should be given in a way that it does not run contrary to the supreme objective. Therefore, we need to follow ethical principles. Education, social relationships, and other human contacts and institutions must also be under that ideal. Political and economic systems must be subordinated to that supreme goal. In fact, one's whole life should be regulated accordingly, if one wants to eliminate mental conflicts and disturbances.

If we have this interpretation of life and sufficient strength to reach the goal, in and through our hopes and aspirations regulated by the higher principles of ethics, then the supreme ideal can be attained, as we have already quoted from the *Gita*. Sri Ramakrishna also gave the same idea to show how one can live in the world a life of the Supreme Reality. He says:

As a boy holding to a post or pillar whirls about it with headlong speed without fear of falling, so perform thy worldly duties, fixing thy hold firmly upon God, and thou shalt be free from danger . . . so be in the world but always remember Him. . . .[16]

In this way we may have the secondary objectives—physical, intellectual, emotional, and esthetic expressions—and not be affected by them. Then, and then alone, can we remove the causes of conflicts and frustrations of the mind. Our behavior becomes harmonious and stable. Nerves become strong. The mind is then full of joy and peace, nay, the supreme goal of human life is reached. Let us remember what Swami Vivekananda says:

Each soul is potentially divine. The goal is to manifest this Divinity within, by controlling nature, external and internal.

[16]*Sayings of Sri Ramakrishna* XXXIV:631.

1*

Do this either by work, or worship, or psychic control, or philosophy, by one or more or all of these—and be free. This is the whole of religion. Doctrines, or dogmas, or rituals, or books, or temples, or forms are but secondary details.[17]

[17] *Works,* I, 257.

APPENDIX

APPENDIX

Vedanta in America[1]

The questions asked by every newcomer who enters a Vedanta temple, lecture room, or center are, quite naturally, almost always the same.

What is this place? What do you do here? What is taught? What is Vedanta? Who is Brahman? What does *Swami* mean?

Vedanta (or Hinduism, as it is usually, but less correctly, called) is the philosophy which has been evolved from the teachings of the Vedas. The Vedas are a collection of ancient Indian scriptures, the oldest religious writings which exist in the world. More generally, the term "Vedanta" includes not only the Vedas themselves but the whole mass of literature which has developed from them, right down to the present day. Vedanta Philosophy is the common basis of India's many sects. Indeed, as will be shown, it demonstrates the essential unity of all religions. It is a sort of philosophical algebra, in terms of which all religious truth can be expressed.

Vedanta teaches three fundamental truths:
1. That Man's real nature is divine.

If, in this universe, there is an underlying Reality, a Godhead, then that Godhead must be omnipresent. If the Godhead is omnipresent, It must be within each one of us and within every creature and object. Therefore Man, in his true nature, is God.

2. That it is the aim of Man's life on earth to unfold and

[1] From a leaflet put out by the Vedanta Society.

manifest this Godhead, which is eternally existent within him, but hidden.

The differences between man and man are only differences in the degree to which the Godhead is manifest. All ethics are merely a means to the end of this divine unfoldment. "Right" action is action which assists the unfoldment of the Godhead within us: "wrong" action is action which hinders that unfoldment. "Good" and "evil" are, therefore, only relative values, and must not be used as an absolute standard by which we judge others. Each individual has an individual problem and an individual path of development. But the goal is the same for all.

Because Man is divine, he has infinite strength and infinite wisdom at his command, if he will use them to uncover his true nature. This nature can be gradually uncovered and known and entered into by means of prayer, meditation and the living of a disciplined life—that is to say, a life which seeks to remove all obstacles to the divine unfoldment. Such obstacles are desire, fear, hatred, possessiveness, vanity and pride. The Vedantist prefers the word "obstacle" to the word "sin" because, if we think of ourselves as sinners and miserable, we forget the Godhead within us and lapse into that mood of doubt, despondency and weakness which is the greatest obstacle of all.

Because the Godhead is within each one of us, Vedanta teaches not merely the brotherhood, but the identity of man with man. It says: "Thou art That." Every soul is your own soul. Every creature is yourself. If you harm anyone, you harm yourself. If you help anyone, you help yourself. Therefore, all feelings of separateness, exclusiveness, intolerance and hatred are not only "wrong," they are the blackest ignorance, because they deny the existence of the omnipresent Godhead, which is One.

3. That truth is universal.

Vedanta accepts all the religions of the world, because it recognizes the same divine inspiration in all. Different religions suit different races, cultures, temperaments. Every religion, like every individual, is involved in a certain measure of ignorance. But Vedanta does not concern itself with that ignorance. It insists on the underlying truth.

Vedanta is impersonal, but it accepts all the great prophets, teachers and sons of God, and all those personal aspects of the Godhead who are worshipped by different religions. According to Vedanta "truth is one; men call it by various names." That truth is what they call Brahman. The Vedantic belief is that all are manifestations of the one Godhead. Accepting all, it does not attempt to make converts. It only seeks to clarify our thought, and thus help us to a truer appreciation of our own religion and its ultimate aim.

Throughout the centuries, Indian Vedanta has produced many great saints and illumined teachers. The latest and in some respects the greatest of these was Sri Ramakrishna (1836-1886).

Sri Ramakrishna spent most of his adult life near Calcutta, living in the grounds of a temple, on the bank of the Ganges. His life expressed, to a greater degree than that of any other teacher, the Vedantic idea of religious universality. After many years of self-discipline and meditation, he reached that realization of identity with the Godhead which Christians call the "mystic union" and Hindus "samadhi." But this did not satisfy him. He then proceeded to test the universality of other religions, including Christianity and Islam. Thus, he was able to say with absolute authority that all religions are true and that the Ultimate Reality can be known by a member of any sect, if his devotion is equal to the task.

Most of Sri Ramakrishna's intimate disciples were young men and boys. After the passing away of their Master they formed a small monastic community which later grew into the Ramakrishna Order. They lived together, or wandered about the country, enduring great hardships and extreme poverty and they realized the highest form of samadhi (superconsciousness) in various ways. Through the Ramakrishna Order the message of the harmony of religions is being spread all over the world.

A Swami is a monk and a religious teacher. He has nothing to do with mystery mongering or occultism or any such expressions of power. He is primarily devoted to God and helps others to do the same. He becomes a monk for the good and happiness of all and he renders loving service to humanity with no racial or religious differentiation.

BIBLIOGRAPHY

Books

ABHEDANANDA, SWAMI. *Christian Science and Vedanta.* San Francisco: Vedanta Ashrama, 1902.

———. *How to Be a Yogi.* Mylapore, Madras: Sri Ramakrishna Math.

———. *Reincarnation.* Mylapore, Madras: Sri Ramakrishna Math.

ALEXANDER, FRANZ. *The Medical Value of Psychoanalysis.* London: Allen & Unwin, 1936.

ALLERS, RUDOLPH. *The Psychology of Character.* London: Sheed & Ward, 1943.

ALLPORT, GORDON W. *Personality, A Psychological Interpretation.* London: Constable, 1937.

Basic Writings of Saint Thomas Aquinas. Vol. I. Edited and annotated by Anton C. Pegis. New York: Random House, Inc., 1945.

Bhagavad-Gita. Translated by Swami Prabhavananda and Christopher Isherwood. Hollywood: The Marcel Rodd Co., 1944. Also, *Srimad-Bhagavad-Gita.* Translated by Swami Swarupananda. 5th ed. Mayavati, Almora, Himalayas: Advaita Ashrama, 1933.

Bhagavatam.

BINGER, CARL. *The Doctor's Job.* New York: W. W. Norton & Co., Inc., 1945.

BORING, EDWIN G. *A History of Experimental Psychology.* London: Appleton, 1929.

BRIGHTMAN, EDGAR S. *A Philosophy of Religion.* New York: Prentice-Hall, Inc., 1940.

———. *The Problem of God.* New York: The Abingdon Press, 1930.

BROWN, WILLIAM. *Science and Personality.* Oxford University Press, 1929.

BUTLER, DON CUTHBERT. *Western Mysticism.* London: Constable & Co., 1922.

Complete Works of Swami Vivekananda, The. Mayavati, Almora, Himalayas: Advaita Ashrama. Vols. I-VII. *Karma Yoga* and *Raja Yoga* (including the *Yoga Aphorisms of Patanjali*), Vol. I; *Jnana Yoga*, Vol. II; *Bhakti Yoga* and *Lectures from Columbo to Almora*, Vol. III; *Inspired Talks*, Vol. VII.

Dhammapada (Sayings of Buddha).

DUTT, D. M. *The Six Ways of Knowing.* London: George Allen & Unwin, Ltd., 1932.

EDDINGTON, A. S. *Nature of the Physical World.* London: Macmillan, 1928.

———. *Philosophy of Physical Science.* London: Macmillan, 1929.

Eternal Companion, The. Hollywood: Vedanta Society of Southern California, 1944.

FADIMAN, CLIFTON (ED.) *I Believe.* New York: Simon & Schuster, 1939.

FREUD, SIGMUND. *Beyond the Pleasure Principle.* London: International Psychoanalytic Press, 1922.

———. *Psychopathology of Everyday Life.* T. Fisher Unwin, Ltd., 1917.

Gospel of Sri Ramakrishna. 2 vols. Mylapore, Madras: Sri Ramakrishna Math, 1930. Also, *The Gospel of Sri Ramakrishna.* Translated by Swami Nikhilananda. New York: Ramakrishna-Vivekananda Center, 1942.

Hatha Yoga Pradipika.

HEIDBREDER, EDNA. *Seven Psychologies.* London: Appleton, 1933.

HENDERSON, D. K., AND GILLESPIE, R. D. *A Textbook of Psychiatry.* London: Oxford University Press, 1937.

HORNEY, KAREN. *Self-Analysis.* London: Kegan Paul, 1942.

JAMES, WILLIAM. "The Energies of Man." *Memories and Studies.* London: Longmans, 1911.

———. *Varieties of Religious Experiences.* London: Longmans, 1929.

JONES, RUFUS M. *Studies in Mystical Religion.* London: Macmillan, 1923.

JUNG, CARL G. *Integration of the Personality.* Translated by Stanley Dell. London: Kegan Paul, 1939.

———. *Modern Man in Search of a Soul.* London: Kegan Paul, 1935.

———. *Psychology and Religion.* New Haven: Yale University Press, 1938.

———. *Psychology of the Unconscious.* London: Kegan Paul, 1931.

KEMPIS, THOMAS À. *The Following of Christ.* New York: Catholic Publishing Co.

LAWRENCE, BROTHER. *The Practice of the Presence of God.* New York: Fleming H. Revell Co., 1895.

LEVINE, ALBERT J. *Current Psychologies.* Cambridge: Sci-Art Publishers, 1940.

Life of St. Teresa of Jesus, The. Autobiography. Translated by David Lewis. London: Thomas Baker, 1924.

Life of Sri Ramakrishna. 3rd ed. Mayavati, Almora, Himalayas: Advaita Ashrama, 1929. Also ROLLAND, ROMAIN. *The Life of Ramakrishna.* Mayavati, Almora, Himalayas: Advaita Ashrama, 1931.

McDOUGALL, WILLIAM. *Outline of Abnormal Psychology.* London: Methuen, 1926.

Meister Eckhart. Translated by Blakney. 2nd ed. New York: Harper & Brothers, 1944.

MAIER, N. R. F., AND SCHNEIRLA, T. C. *Principles of Animal Psychology.* New York: McGraw-Hill Book Co., 1935.

MENNINGER, KARL A. *Love Against Hatred.* New York: Harcourt, Brace & Co., Inc., 1942.

———. *Man Against Himself.* New York: Harcourt, Brace & Co., Inc., 1938.

MÜLLER-FREINFELS, RICHARD. *Evolution of Modern Psychology.* Translated by W. Béran Wolfe. New Haven: Yale University Press, 1935.

NEW TESTAMENT. *Holy Bible.* Matthew, Mark, Romans, and II Corinthians.

OTTO, RUDOLF. *Mysticism East and West.* Translated by Bertha L. Bracey and Richenda C. Payne. London: Macmillan, 1932.

———. *The Idea of the Holy.* Translated by John W. Harvey. London: Humphrey Milford, Oxford University Press, 1925.

PATANJALI. *Yoga Aphorisms.*

PRATT, JAMES BISSELL. *The Religious Consciousness.* New York: Macmillan Co., 1920.

RHINE, JOSEPH BANKS, AND OTHERS. *Extrasensory Perceptions after Sixty Years.* London: Faber, 1940.

————. *New Frontiers of the Mind.* London: Faber, 1937.

ROGERS, CARL R. *Counseling and Psychotherapy.* Boston: Houghton Mifflin Co., 1942.

SARADANANDA, SWAMI. *Sri Sri Ramakrishna Lilaprasanga.* Vol. II, *Sadhaka Bhava.* Calcutta: Udbohan Office.

Sayings of Sri Ramakrishna. Mylapore, Madras: Sri Ramakrishna Math, 1925.

SCHOLEM, GERSHOM G. *Major Trends in Jewish Mysticism.* Jerusalem: Schoken Publishing House, 1941.

SEAL, SIR B. N. *The Positive Sciences of the Ancient Hindus.* London: Longmans, 1915.

SOROKIN, PITIRIM A. *The Crisis of Our Age.* New York: E. P. Dutton & Co., Inc., 1942.

Spiritual Teachings of Swami Brahmananda. 2nd ed. Mylapore, Madras: Sri Ramakrishna Math, 1933.

SPRANGER, EDUARD. *Types of Man.* New York: G. E. Stechert & Co., 1928.

STROMBERG, GUSTAF. *The Soul of the Universe.* Philadelphia: David McKay Co., 1940.

SUTRAS. Narada, *Bhakti Sutra; Yoga Sutra;* and *Vedanta (Brahma) Sutra.*

Theologia Germanica. Translated by Susanna Winkworth. London: Macmillan & Co., 1874.

THOMAS, WILLIAM I., AND ZNANIECKI, FLORIAN. *The Polish Peasant in Europe and America.* Vol. III, *Life Record of an Immigrant.* Boston: Richard G. Badger, The Gorham Press, 1919.

UNDERHILL, EVELYN. *Mysticism.* 7th ed. London: Methuen & Co., Ltd., 1918.

UPANISHADS. *Chhandagya Upanishad; Katha Upanishad; Kena Upanishad; Mandukya Upanishad; Svetasvatra Upanishad; Taittiriya Upanishad,* Vol. VII, *Brahmananda Valli;* and Sri Sankaracharya, *Vivekachudamani.*

Vedanta Paribhasa.

Vida de La Santa Madre Terasa de Jesus, La (1881). Vol. I (in D. Vicinti de Fuenti, *Abras de Santa Terasa de Jesus*).

Vivarana Prameya Samgraha.

WATSON, JOHN B. *Behaviorism.* London: Kegan Paul.

Way of Perfection. London: Thomas Baker, 1935.

WOODWORTH, ROBERT S. *Contemporary Schools of Psychology.* New York: The Ronald Press Co., 1931.

Yoga. Mayavati, Almora, Himalayas: Advaita Ashrama; and New York: Ramakrishna-Vedanta Society. The different systems of *yoga* are separately published in Mayavati, Almora, Himalayas by the Advaita Ashrama; and in New York by the Ramakrishna-Vedanta Society.

Articles

ALLPORT, GORDON W. "The Psychology of Participation," *The Psychological Review*, LII (May, 1945), 117-31.

CARLSON, A. J. "Science and the Supernatural," *Scientific Monthly*, LIX (August, 1944), 85-95.

HOCKING, W. E. "Mind and Near-Mind," *Proceedings of the Sixth International Congress of Philosophy*, Edited by Edgar Sheffield Brightman. New York: Longmans, Green & Co., 1927, pp. 203 and 215.

HUNT, J. McV. "Social Conflict in Psychosis," *The American Journal of Orthopsychiatry*, VIII (January, 1938).

"Importance of Introducing Psychiatry into General Internship, The," *Journal of the American Medical Association*, CII (1934), 982-86 and 1231-32.

PRATT, JOSEPH H. *The Influence of Emotions in the Causation and Cure of Psychoneuroses*. Philadelphia: J. B. Lippincott Co., 1934. Reprinted from *International Clinics*, Vol. IV, Series 44.

Index